Step by Step in EMERGENCY RADIOLOGY

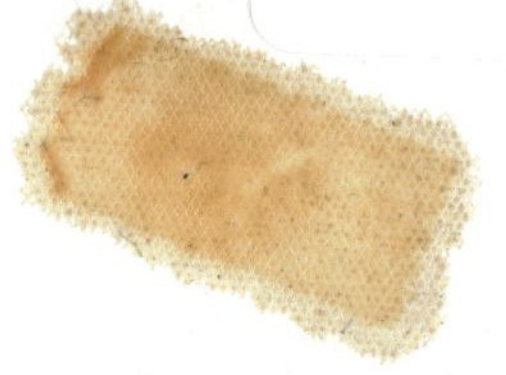

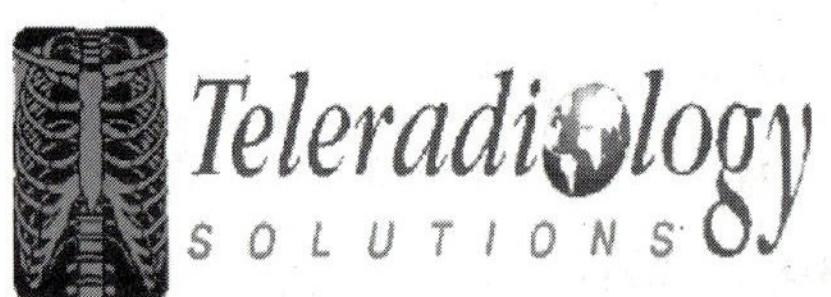

CD CONTENTS

Interesting Cases

Step by Step in EMERGENCY RADIOLOGY

Helical CT in Acute Abdomen

Series Editor

Arjun Kalyanpur MD ABR
Chief Radiologist
Teleradiology Solutions

Textbook Editors

Arjun Kalyanpur MD ABR
Chief Radiologist
Teleradiology Solutions

Jagdish Singh DNB DMRD
Consultant Radiologist
Teleradiology Solutions

Authors

Jagdish Singh DNB DMRD
Consultant Radiologist
Teleradiology Solutions

Vandana Verma Marwah MD
Consultant Radiologist
Teleradiology Solutions

Ravi Kumar MD
Consultant Radiologist
Teleradiology Solutions

Srinivas M DNB DMRD
Consultant Radiologist
Teleradiology Solutions

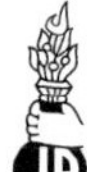

JAYPEE BROTHERS
MEDICAL PUBLISHERS (P) LTD
New Delhi

Published by

Jitendar P Vij
Jaypee Brothers Medical Publishers (P) Ltd
EMCA House, 23/23B Ansari Road, Daryaganj
New Delhi 110 002, India
Phones: +91-11-23272143, +91-11-23272703, +91-11-23282021, +91-11-23245672
Fax: +91-11-23276490, +91-11-23245683 e-mail: jaypee@jaypeebrothers.com
Visit our website: www.jaypeebrothers.com

Branches

- 2/B Akruti Society, Jodhpur Gam Road, Satellite, **Ahmedabad** 380 015,
Phone: +91-079-30988717, +91-079-26926233
- 202 Batavia Chambers, 8 Kumara Krupa Road, Kumara Park East,
Bangalore 560 001, Phones: +91-80-22285971, +91-80-22382956, +91-80-30614073
Tele Fax: +91-80-22281761 e-mail: jaypeemedpubbgl@eth.net
- 282 IIIrd Floor, Khaleel Shirazi Estate, Fountain Plaza
Pantheon Road, **Chennai** 600 008, Phones: +91-44-28262665, +91-44-28269897
Fax: +91-44-28262331 e-mail: jpchen@eth.net
- 4-2-1067/1-3, Ist Floor, Balaji Building, Ramkote
Cross Road, **Hyderabad** 500 095, Phones: +91-40-55610020, +91-40-24758498
Fax: +91-40-24758499 e-mail: jpmedpub@rediffmail.com
- 1A Indian Mirror Street, Wellington Square, **Kolkata** 700 013,
Phones: +91-33-22456075, +91-33-22451926 Fax: +91-33-22456075
e-mail: jpbcal@cal.vsnl.net.in
- 106 Amit Industrial Estate, 61 Dr SS Rao Road, Near MGM Hospital
Parel, **Mumbai** 400 012, Phones: +91-22-24124863, +91-22-24104532, +91-22-30926896
Fax: +91-22-24160828 e-mail: jpmedpub@bom7.vsnl.net.in
e-mail: jpmedpub@bom7.vsnl.net.in
- "KAMALPUSHPA", 38 Reshimbag, Opp. Mohota Science College, Umred Road
Nagpur 440 009, Phones: +91-712-3945220, +91-712-2704275
e-mail: jpnagpur@rediffmail.com

Step by Step in Emergency Radiology

First Edition: **2006**

ISBN 81-8061-803-X

Typeset at JPBMP typesetting unit
Printed at Gopsons Paper Ltd, Noida

PREFACE

Emergency Radiology in India represents an idea whose time has come. Quality emergency medical services are the crying need of the hour. In all other respects, our country has evolved rapidly in recent years in terms of medical care delivery, exemplified in the radiology setting by the number of recent installations of helical and multidetector-row CT scanners throughout the country. The anatomy of the abdomen and pelvis is revealed in startling detail to us with multiplanar CT imaging, allowing us to diagnose pathology with a high degree of sensitivity and accuracy.

Another paradigm shift that is taking place is the switch to reading studies on monitors rather than on hard copy film. Given economic constraints, reading off film is inherently unsafe as in an effort to cut costs, the minimum possible number of window settings is typically presented to the radiologist. Soft copy review has opened up the Pandora's Box (i.e. the abdomen/pelvis) to radiologists throughout the country. When I began residency training in the US in the early 90s I was amazed at the amount of mesenteric pathology that was revealed to me just by virtue of having the luxury of being able to window and level to my heart's desire. One of the shortcomings of radiologic practice and training in India at the time was the lack of emphasis on the CT imaging of mesenteric disease. Although I learned a great deal during my residency training in New Delhi, I credit my US training with giving me the ability to spot tiny amounts of mesenteric fluid and air and the subtlest of 'fat stranding' and to use these findings as a clue/pointer to make the actual diagnosis. It is these signs/findings that we have attempted to highlight in this book.

The imaging equipment and workstations are now in place, now it is up to us as radiologists to train ourselves in the art and science of emergency abdominal imaging to meet the challenges that our patients present to us. This book is written with the goal of increasing the awareness of our community to our potential as radiologists in effecting enhanced patient care. It represents the cumulative results of three years of emergency imaging and a lot of hard work by our team at Teleradiology Solutions, spearheaded by Dr Jagdish Singh. We hope you enjoy it. If even a single patient benefits from your perusal of it, our purpose is fulfilled.

Arjun Kalyanpur

ACKNOWLEDGEMENTS

Dr Arjun Kalyanpur and Dr Sunita Maheswari for their motivation and guidance

Neetu Jagdish Singh and Dr. Deepa Ravikumar for helping in writing the manuscript

Akram Pervez and Munnawar Pasha, medical transcriptionists, Teleradiology Solutions, for typing out the written text

Siddharth Ghosh, medical transcriptionist, Teleradiology Solutions for helping in downloading and printing the material needed for writing the book

Family members of the authors for their moral support.

All our colleagues at Teleradiology Solutions for their support.

CONTENTS

CHAPTER 1

Introduction

Acute abdomen is a clinical condition characterized by sudden onset of severe abdominal pain requiring immediate medical or surgical treatment.[1]

Early and accurate diagnosis is essential to minimize morbidity and mortality. The clinical analysis of acute abdomen is challenging because the clinical symptoms, physical signs and laboratory findings are not always diagnostic and are often nonspecific. Delay in diagnosis results in severe complications, increased hospital stay and postoperative complications. Also the spectrum of differential diagnosis is numerous ranging from minor self-limiting disorders to catastrophic conditions requiring immediate operation and intervention.[2]

Imaging plays a vital role[3] in acute and early diagnosis helps prevent complications, surgical interventions and hospital cost, negative laparotomies, reduced cost and hospital stay.

Plain film radiography and sonography form the initial mode of investigation—plain films can be used to detect free air or pattern of bowel gas distribution or abnormal calcification, however they are limited in specificity.

Although sonography[4] is well-established in evaluation of gallbladder disorders in children and women of child-bearing age, it is limited by the presence of bowel gas, body habitus, is operative dependent and difficult for the clinicians to understand

Helical CT is fast-evolving[5-7] as an effective technique for evaluation of acute abdomen. CT is rapid, less-invasive, not affected by bowel gas or abdominal fat. It can cover a wide range of abnormalities including gut, mesentery, omentum, peritoneum and retroperitoneal pathologies. Further more, 3-dimensional depictions helps clinicians understand the pathology better and help management.

The subsequent chapters will describe the practical approach and salient features of CT in acute abdominal disorders.

REFERENCES

1. Silen W. Cope's early diagnosis of the acute abdomen, 19th ed. New York: Oxford University Press 1996.
2. Trott AT, Lucas RH. Acute abdominal pain. In: Rose P, ed. Emergency medicine, 4th ed. St Louis Mosby 1998 : 1888-1903.
3. Sturman MF. Medical Imaging in acute abdominal pain Compr Ther 1991; 170: 361-71.
4. Puylaert JBCM, Vanderzant FM, Rjke AM. Sonography and the acute abdomen practical considerations. AJR 1997: 168:179-86.
5. Malone AJ. Unenhanced CT in the evaluation of the acute abdomen. Semin Ultrasound CT MR 1996; 205: 43-7.
6. Siewert B. Raptspoulos V, Mueller MF, Rosen MP, Steer M. Impact of CT on diagnosis and management of acute abdomen in patients initially treated without surgery. AJR 1997; 168: 173-8.
7. Novelline RA, Rhea JT, Rao PM, Stuk JL. Helical CT in emergency radiology. Radiology 1999; 213: 321-39.

Chapter 2

Helical CT Technique and Protocols

INTRODUCTION

There are a variety of patient preparation and CT protocols to study the diverse cause of acute abdomen. The selection of the protocols depends on the clinical indication and the likely diagnosis. Also the examination may be a focused or general survey including the abdomen and pelvis.[1] It is ideal to obtain a general survey examination covering the entire abdomen and pelvis to cover a broad range of differential diagnosis. Moreover with the advent of helical and particularly multidetector CT, the time taken for examinations is much decreased, allowing for coverage of the entire abdomen and pelvis in a single breath-hold.

Scans are obtained from the level of the diaphragm to the symphysis pubis. The scan parameters include collimation of 5 to 7 mm, thinner sections for an area of interest, a pitch of 1.0 to 1.5.

Scan can be done with or without contrast depending on the indications. Plain scans are used best for renal, ureteric, CBD stones or detection of appendicoliths.

Oral contrast may be employed in bowel pathologies, in appendicitis ,to differentiate bowel loops from fluid collection or abscesses. Delayed rescans after 2 to 3 hours may be necessary if the distal small bowel or colon remain unopacified/underdistended on the initial series. Rectal contrast increases the accuracy of appendix visualization as well as colonic wall thickening in colitis and diverticulitis.[2]

Ideally, 800 to 1000 ml of a diluted water soluble contrast material may be given 1 hour before scanning.

Intravenous contrast is helpful in the diagnosis of bowel ischemia, vascular thrombosis, to detect inflammatory mural changes in appendicitis, cholecystitis, diverticulitis, Crohn's disease, in detection of abscesses, or demonstrating active contrast extravasation in ruptured aneurysms. Between 100 and 125 ml of nonionic intravenous contrast material may be injected at the rate of 3 ml/sec. Scans both in the arterial and delayed phase should be obtained.

We recommend that CT be performed with oral and intravenous contrast in all cases, unless intravenous contrast is specifically contraindicated, or in the case of suspected nephroureterolithiasis (Table 2.1).

TABLE 2.1

Scan Protocol	*Contrast*	*Indication*
I	No contrast	Best for renal, ureteral, CBD calculi, appendicoliths
II	Oral/Rectal	Colon and appendix.
III	Oral/Rectal/IV	Colon, appendix, bowel ischemia, abscesses

REFERENCES

1. Mindelzun RE, Jeffrey RB. The acute abdomen: current CT imaging techniques. Semin Ultrasound CT MR 1999; 20: 63-7.
2. Rao PM. Rhea JT, Novelline RA, Mostafavi A, Laurason JN, MC Cabe CT. Helical CT scanning with contrast material administered only through the colon for imaging suspected appendicitis. AJR 1997; 169: 1275-80.

CHAPTER 3

Common Acute Abdominal Pathologies

APPENDICITIS

Appendicitis is the commonest abdominal emergency. The classic presentation is with pain, vomiting and fever with rebound tenderness in the right lower abdomen. However clinical evaluation is always not diagnostic, as the presentation is oftern nonspecific. Numerous other conditions mimic appendicitis and hence clinical evaluation may be equivocal. Also delay in diagnosis may result in perforation and complication. The reported rate of perforation is 20% in the literature.[1, 2] Imaging plays an important role in early diagnosis and management.

Plain radiographs are limited in utility and the signs are nonspecific. Ultrasound is an effective tool in the evaluation of appendicitis. It is of proven value in children and early stages. However, it is operator-dependent, limited by bowel gas and less-effective in diagnosis of perforation and its sequelae.

CT has evolved as an effective tool in the evaluation of appendicitis. It is highly-sensitive and specific.[3] It can detect the early, subtle inflamed appendix, help detect perforation and its complications and provide alternative diagnoses in negative cases.

NORMAL APPEARANCE ON CT AND PATHOLOGY

The normal appendix is often easily identified on CT scans of the abdomen. It appears as a thinwalled tubular structure arising from the cecum between the ileocecal

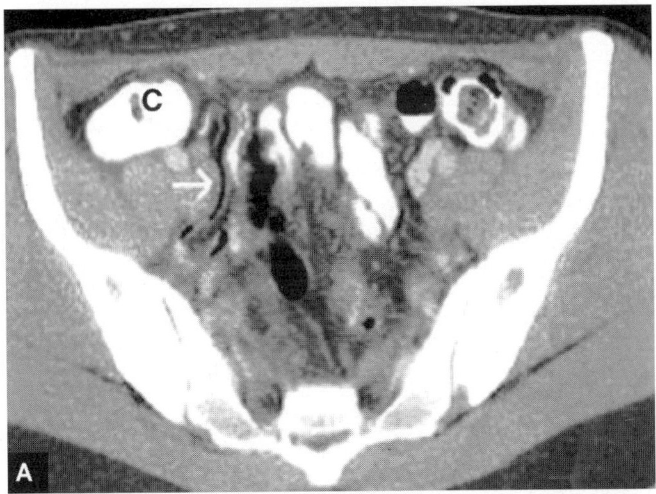

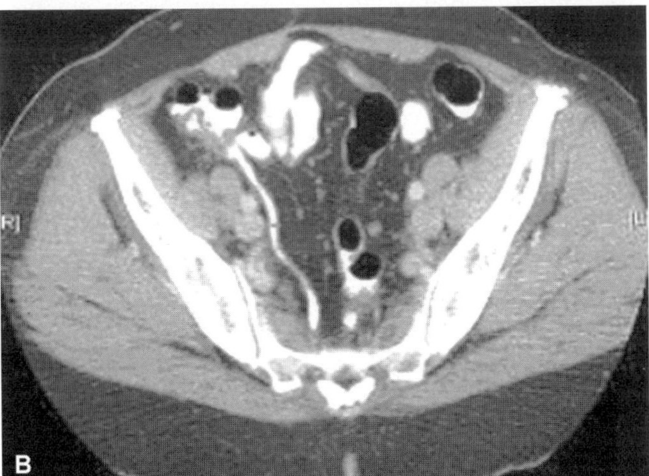

FIGURES 3.1A and B: Normal appearance of appendix on CT. (A) Normal air-filled appendix (arrow). (B) Normal contrast-filled appendix with its tip in the pelvis

valve and cecal tip. It may be air filled or contrast filled (Figure 3.1). The location is variable and can be in the pelvis, or retrocecal.[4] Ideally, it is helpful to trace the ileocecal valve and search for the appendix. It can vary from 5-20 cm. The normal appendix measures 5-6 mm in transverse dimension on CT. It is normally surrounded by homogeneous low attenuation fat. Thinner sections of 5 mm or less help in better visualization of the appendix.[5,6] Also administration of oral/rectal/IV contrast increases the probability of identification of the appendix.

The etiology and pathogenesis of appendicitis is not clear. However, mechanical obstruction of the appendiceal lumen, either because of fecal stasis, peritoneal adhesions or mural lymphoid hyperplasia may have a role. Inflammation results in accumulation of fluid, appendiceal dilatation, and in later stages ischemia and eventually perforation with abscess formation.

CT FEATURES OF APPENDICITIS AND ITS COMPLICATION

CT FEATURES OF EARLY APPENDICITIS

The diagnostic CT signs of early acute appendicitis are identification of an abnormal appendix.

1. Fluid-filled thickened appendix more than (7 mm) in transverse diameter, with a circumferentially enhancing wall

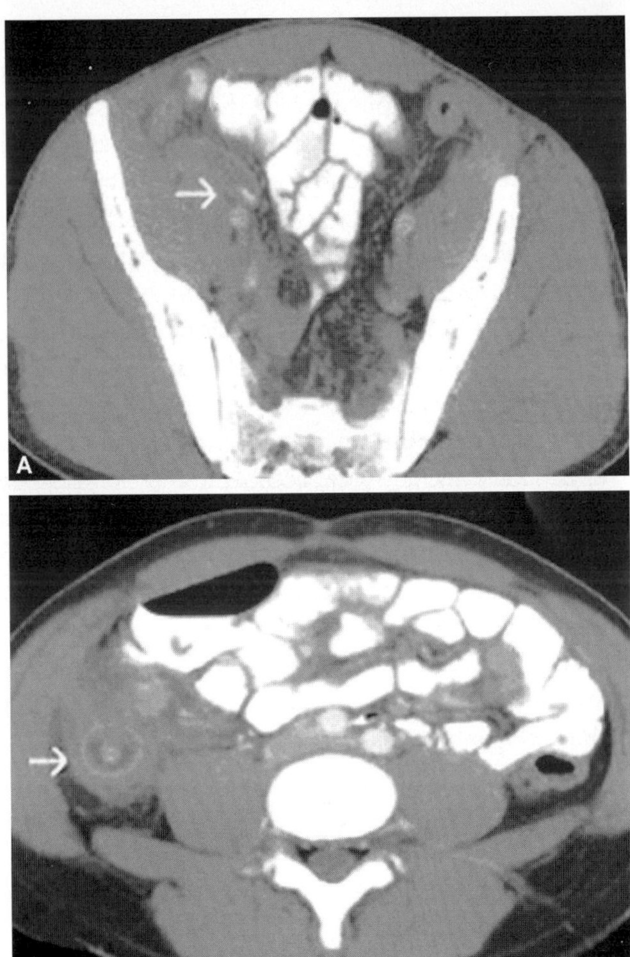

FIGURES 3.2A and B: Abnormal appendix on CT. (A) Dilated, fluid-filled appendix (arrow) with enhancing wall and an appendicolith. (B) Markedly thickened appendix with an appendicolith (arrow) and extensive periappendiceal stranding

2. Fluid-filled appendix with or without an appendicolith associated with pericecal inflammatory stranding (Figure 3.2). Periappendiceal stranding is present in 98%[7-9] of patients with acute appendicitis. The presence of an appendicolith alone without surrounding stranding, or presence of pericecal stranding without definite identification of an abnormal appendix are suspicious for acute appendicitis but not diagnostic,[8, 9] because many other conditions such as Crohn's disease, or cecal diverticulitis may demonstrate inflammatory changes.
3. Other CT findings that may be suggestive of acute appendicitis include focal cecal apical thickening and the 'arrowhead sign".[10] The arrowhead sign (Figure 3.3) has been defined as an arrowhead-shaped collection of contrast material in the cecum that points to the occluded appendiceal lumen. The arrowhead sign is thought to arise when the walls of the cecal apex become thickened, resulting in a triangular-shaped space that becomes filled with contrast material. This secondary sign has high specificity[10] and may be helpful to establish the diagnosis in equivocal cases.
4. Sometimes the inflammation of the appendix may be localized to the distal aspect. Therefore, it is important to try to localize the entire length of the appendix on CT. The CT features of distal appendicitis[11] are diagnosed when CT shows signs of appendicitis that involve the distal aspect of appendix, with a normal

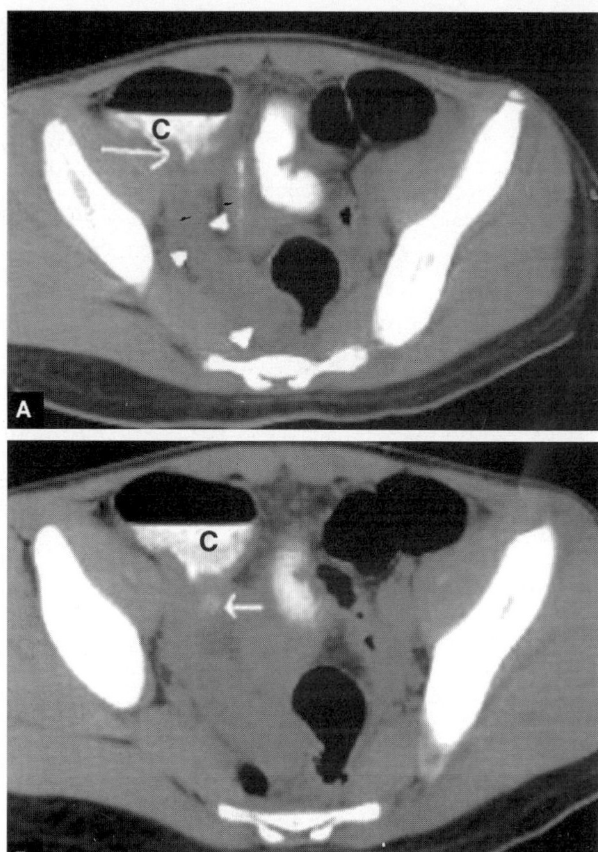

FIGURES 3.3A and B: CT "arrowhead sign". (A) CT scan with oral contrast shows an arrow-shaped collection of contrast at the cecal base (long arrow) with tubular soft tissue density in the pelvis (arrowheads). (B) An appendicolith is seen at the cecal base (long arrow), The "arrowhead sign" has been defined as an arrowhead-shaped collection of contrast material in the cecum that points to the occluded appendiceal lumen. The arrowhead sign is thought to arise when the walls of the cecal apex become thickened, resulting in a triangular-shaped space that becomes filled with contrast material

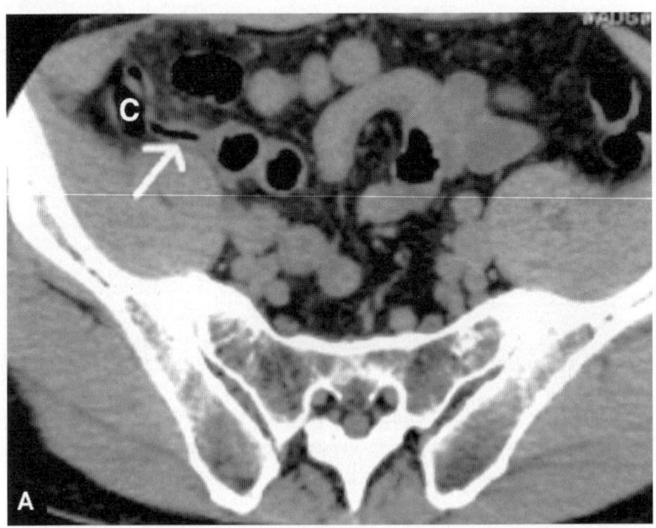

3.4A

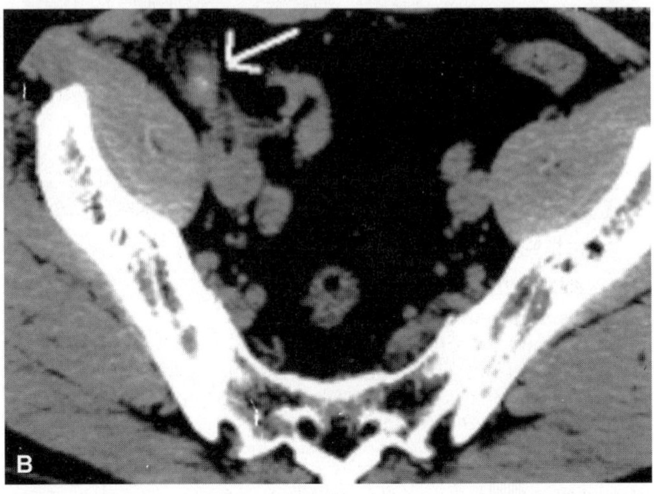

3.4B

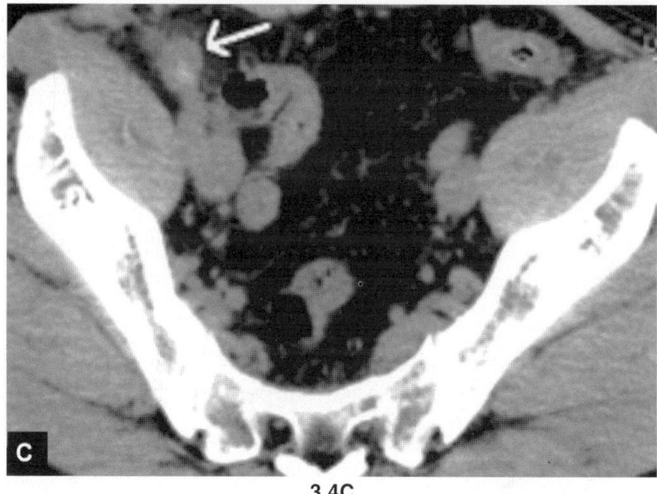

3.4C

FIGURES 3.4A to C: Patient presented with right lower quadrant pain and suspected appendicitis. (A) The proximal appendix is air filled and is within normal limits (arrow). (B) There is an appendicolith (arrow) within the mid-appendicular lumen. (C) The distal appendix is thickened (arrow) with surrounding periappendiceal fat stranding consistent with acute distal appendicitis

proximal appendix and cecal apex (Figure 3.4). Very often an obstructing appendicolith can be identified at the transition point between the normal and abnormal appendix

CT FEATURES OF PERFORATED APPENDIX AND ITS COMPLICATIONS

If the diagnosis is delayed, inflammation leads to progressive appendiceal dilatation, and in later stages ischemia and eventually perforation resulting in an inflammation or phlegmon like mass, and ultimately in abscess formation. The appendix itself may be difficult to identify in these situations.

Perforated appendicitis is usually associated with pericecal phlegmon or abscess formation. Intravenous contrast may be useful in cases of perforation by demonstrating a breech in the appendiceal wall (Figure 3.5). If the abnormal appendix is not seen, identifying an appendicolith with a periappendiceal phlegmon or abscess can help to diagnose appendicitis.

The other findings associated with perforation include extraluminal air, marked ileocecal wall thickening, peritonitis and secondary small bowel obstruction.

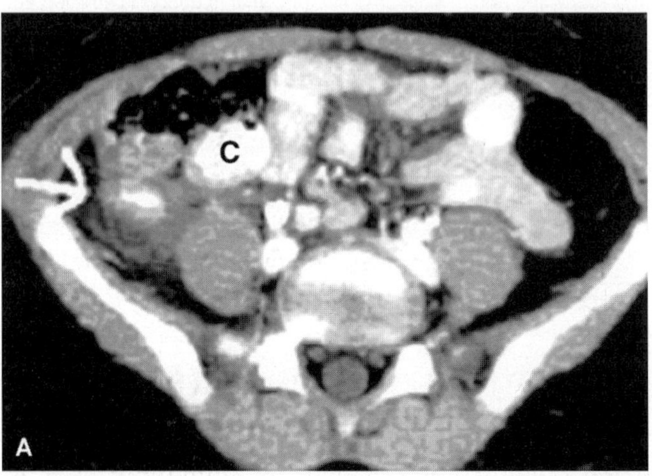

3.5A

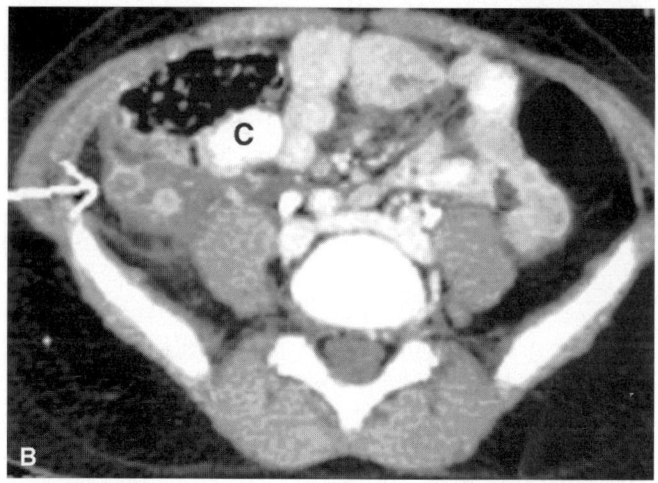

3.5B

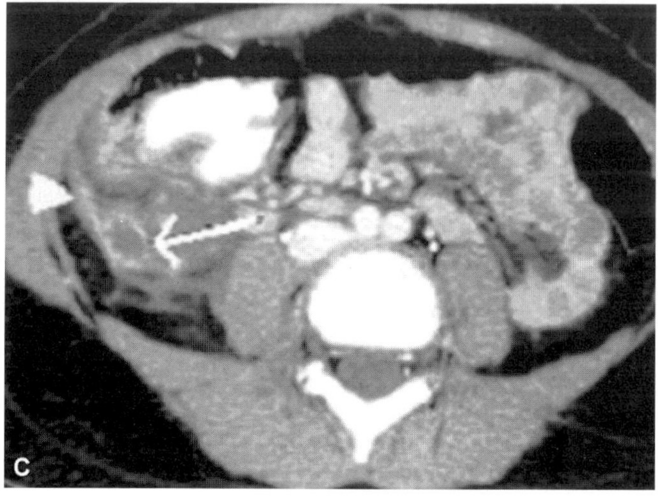

3.5C

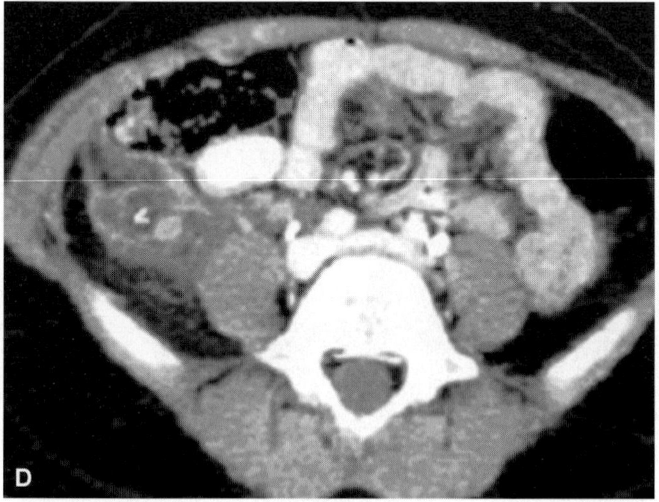

3.5D

FIGURES 3.5A to D: Acute perforated appendicitis. (A) axial scan with oral and intravenous contrast demonstrates thickened base of the appendix (arrow) with periappendiceal stranding. (B) Contrast CT shows a dilated appendix with enhancing walls (arrows) and surrounding fat stranding. (C) Inflamed appendix (arrow) and associated enhancement of the peritoneal lining (arrow head). (D) Contrast enhanced CT demonstrates a disruption in the wall of the distal appendix (small arrow) with associated periappendiceal fat stranding consistent with perforated appendix.C= cecum.

DIFFERENTIAL DIAGNOSIS FOR APPENDICITIS

Various other acute intra-abdominal conditions can mimic acute appendicitis and include cecal diverticulitis (Figure 3.6). Crohn's disease (Figure 3.7), ureteric calculi, Meckel's diverticulitis, ovarian disease, and epiploic appendagitis. CT is helpful in identifying a normal appendix and also

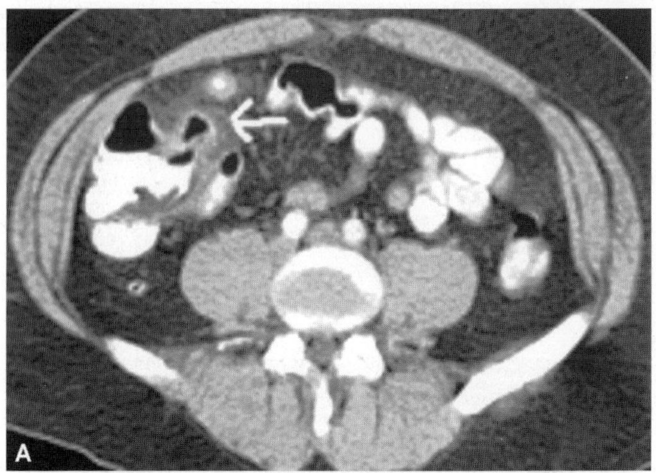

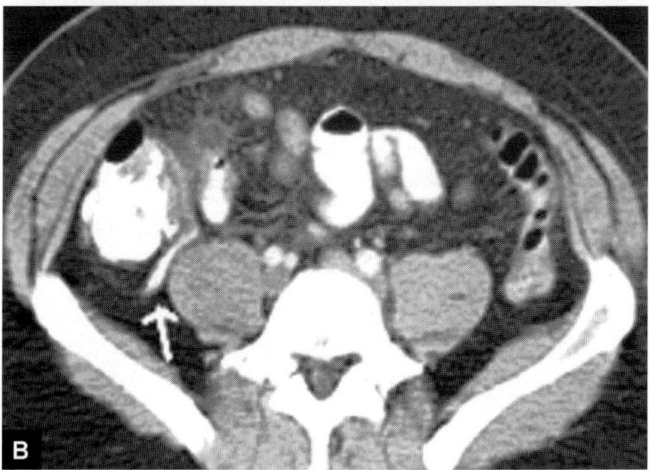

FIGURES 3.6A and B: Patient presented with right lower quadrant pain and suspected appendicitis. (A) axial scan with oral and intravenous contrast showing a cecal diverticulum with thickened walls and surrounding mesenteric fat stranding (arrow). (B) The appendix is contrast-filled and appears within normal limits (long arrow).

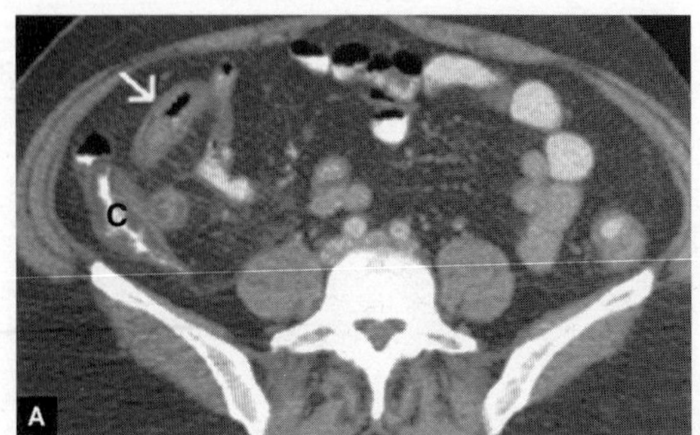

3.7A

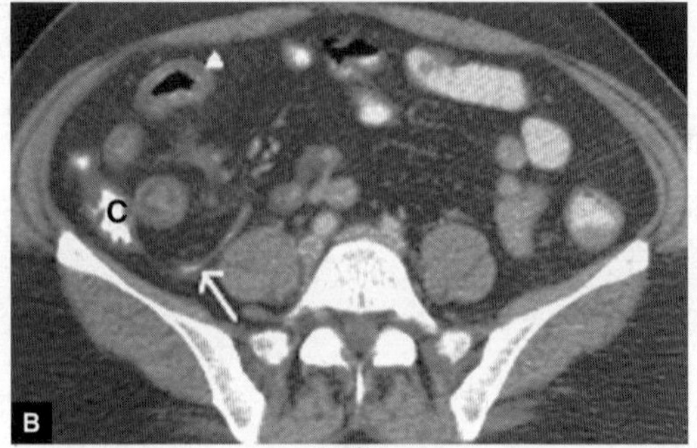

3.7B

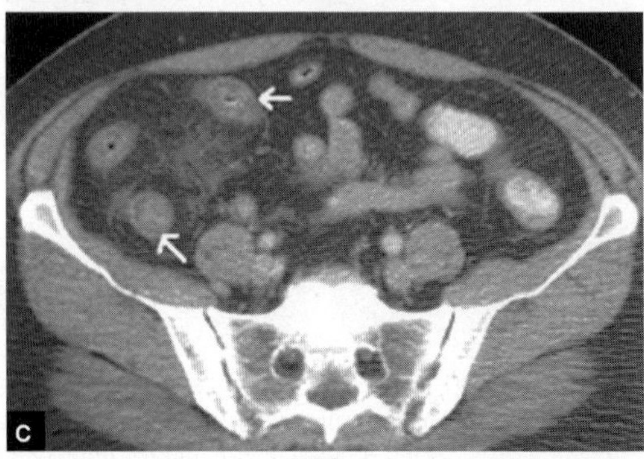

3.7C

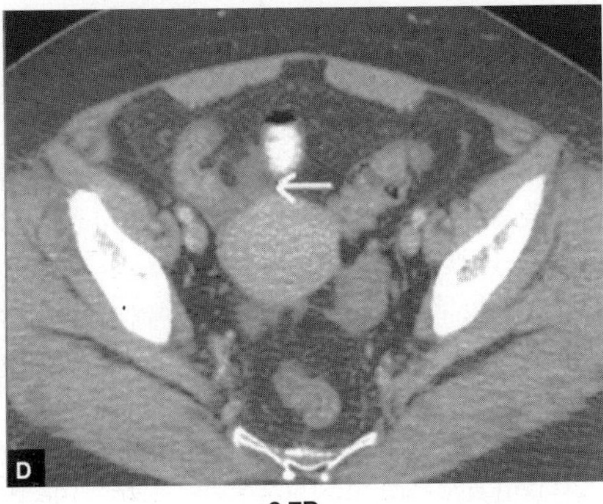

3.7D

FIGURES 3.7A to D: Patient with right lower quadrant pain and suspected appendicitis. (A) Thickened loop of small bowel in the right lower quadrant (arrow), C= cecum. (B) Normal contrast filled appendix (long arrow), with thickened loops of distal ileum (arrowhead). (C,D) Thickened distal small bowel loops (small arrows) with mesenteric fat stranding and minimal free fluid (long arrow), consistent with ileitis

identifying the alternate causes that mimic appendicitis.[12,13]

Conclusion

Acute appendicitis is a common clinical entity with variable clinical presentation.. Helical CT is highly beneficial in the investigation of acute appendicitis, in the identification of an abnormally-located appendix, in the preoperative management of complications and may provide alternative diagnosis in negative cases. The various CT findings and signs described above help in prompt diagnosis and early management.

DIVERTICULITIS

Diverticulitis is a common condition in the west occurring in 10 to 25% of patients with known diverticulosis.[14] With the changing dietary habits, it is not uncommon in our country . Diverticuli are common in the sigmoid, although they can occur throughout the colon.

Patients usually present with left lower quadrant pain, fever, and leucocytosis. Clinical misdiagnosis rate ranges from 34 to 67%.[15]

CT is an ideal imaging technique for diagnosing diverticulitis. It can confirm the diagnosis, detect the presence of complications (abscess, perforation), guide for percutaneous aspiration, or exclude diverticulitis and provide an alternative diagnosis.

On CT, diverticuli appear as small, air or contrast-filled outpouchings of the colonic wall, most abundant in the sigmoid colon (Figure 3.8).

TECHNIQUE AND PROTOCOL

For evaluating suspected diverticulitis, the use of thinner 5 mm sections is recommended. Oral/rectal contrast can be used. When oral contrast is used, scanning should be delayed till 2 hours following completion of contrast ingestion to ensure optimal colonic opacification/ distension. Rectal contrast should be administered cautiously using a flexible catheter to avoid perforating an acutely inflamed colon. Intravenous contrast can be helpful in detecting abscess.

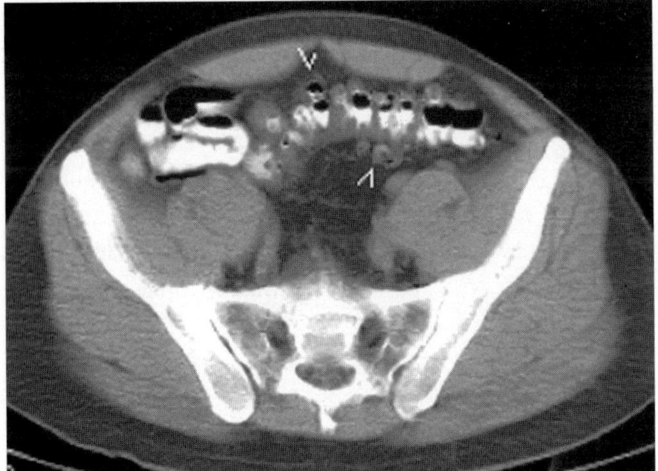

FIGURE 3.8: Normal diverticulosis on CT. Axial scan with oral contrast in the colon showing small air or contrast-filled out pouchings from the sigmoid colon (small arrows) representing the diverticuli

CT FEATURES OF DIVERTICULITIS

The CT hallmark of diverticulitis are inflammatory changes in the pericolonic fat seen in 98%.[16] In milder cases, there is increased haziness of pericolonic fat, fascial thickening, minimal fluid in the gutters and asymmetric colonic wall thickening.[17]

In severe cases there may be marked wall thickening (Figure 3.9), phlegmon or frank abscess formation (Figure 3.10). Perforation may be contained with adjacent extraluminal loculi of air or may be frank, in which case free intraperitoneal air can be detected in distant locations. Other complications of diverticulitis include large or small bowel obstruction (Figure 3.11) or the formation of fistulas.

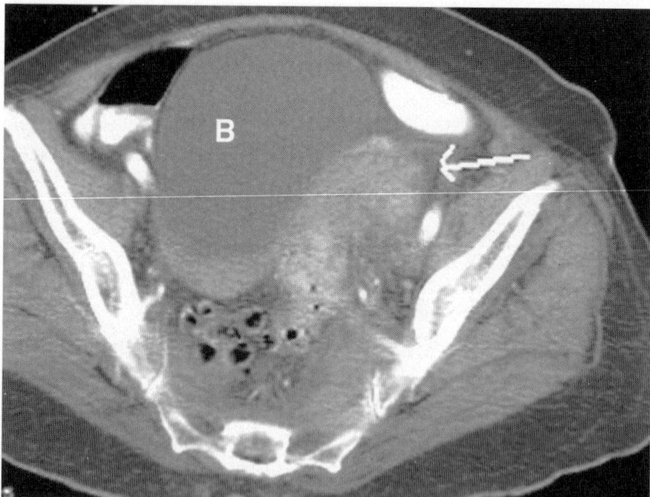

FIGURE 3.9: Patient with pelvic pain and fever. Axial scan showing multiple sigmoid diverticuli with focal wall thickening and surrounding stranding (arrow) suggestive of diverticulitis

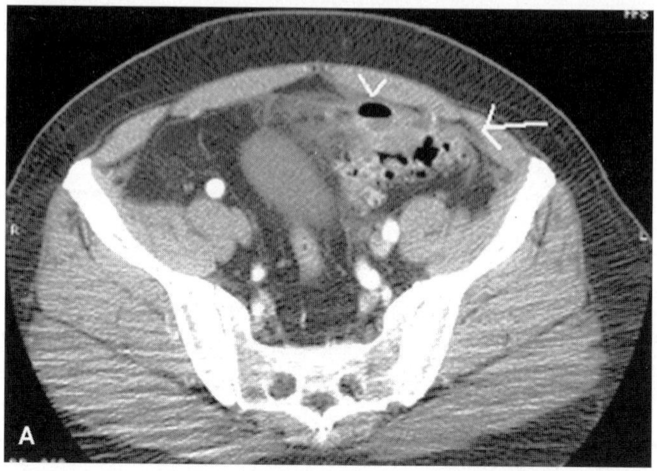

3.10A

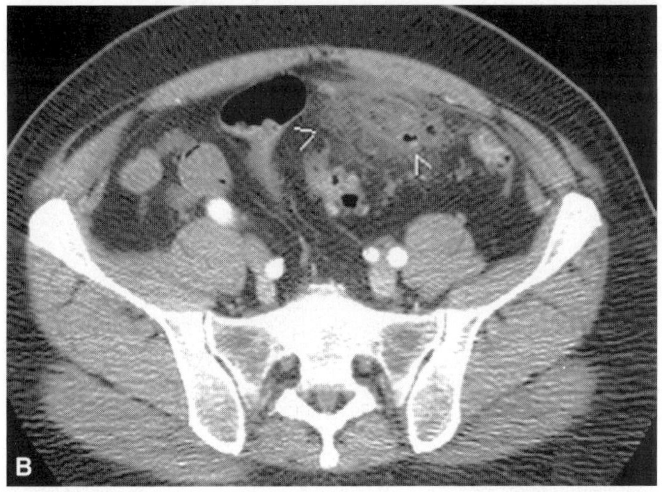

3.10B

FIGURES 3.10A and B: Patient with acute abdominal pain and suspected diverticulitis. (A) Axial scan showing thickened sigmoid colon, adjacent fat stranding (large arrow) and associated pericolonic abscess (small arrow). (B) Extensive mesenteric stranding and extraluminal loculi of air (small arrows)

Occasionally, diverticulitis involves the right colon and cecum and can mimic appendicitis or cholecystitis.

CT findings of right-sided diverticulitis consists of pericolonic inflammatory change, asymmetric wall thickening and the presence of a diverticulum (Figure 3.12). Usually the normal appendix is seen. If the appendix is not seen, differential diagnosis includes appendicitis, epiploic appendagitis, and focal colitis.

A perforated carcinoma of the sigmoid colon can mimic sigmoid diverticulitis. Features suggestive of diverticulitis include asymmetric thickening less than 1 cm,

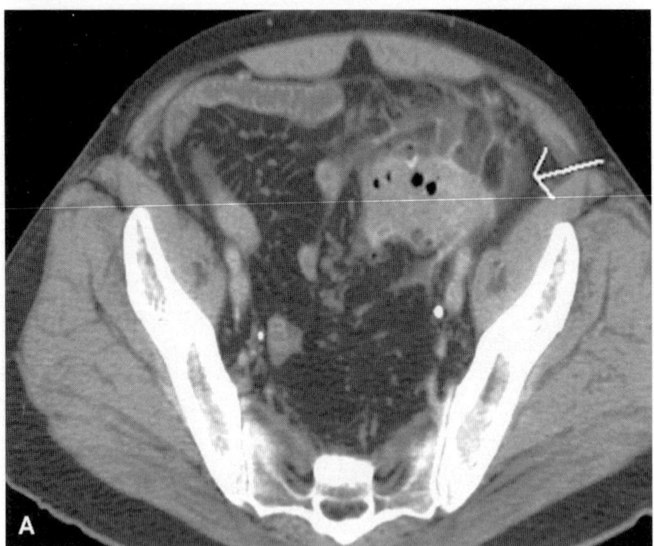

3.11A

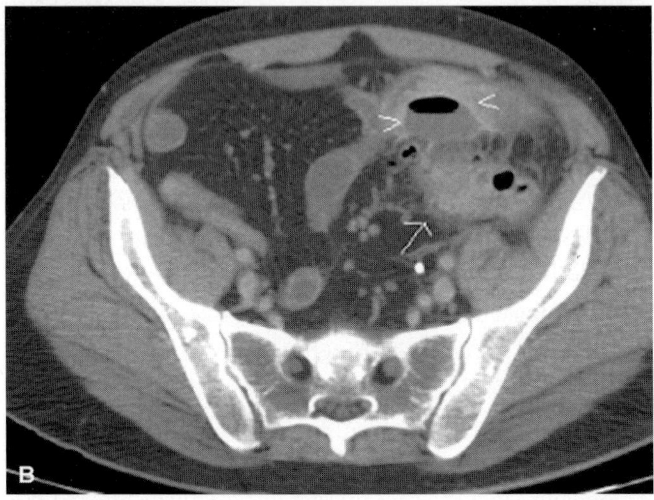

3.11B

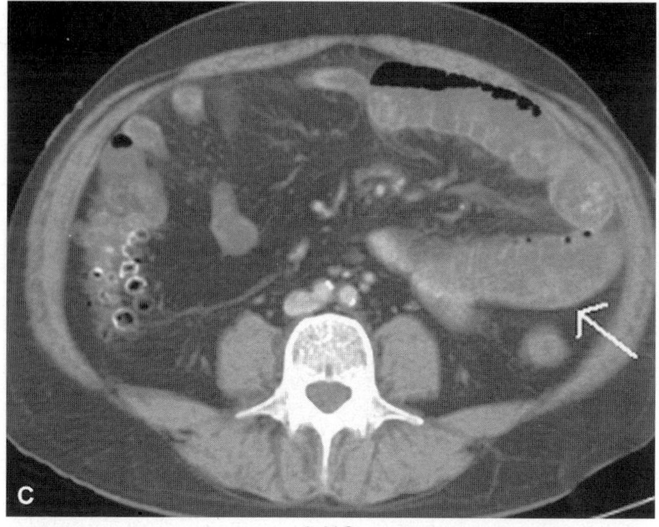

3.11C

FIGURES 3.11A to C: Patient with severe acute abdominal pain and distension (A,B) Perforated sigmoid diverticulitis (large arrow) with abscess (small arrows) compressing a segment of small bowel. (C) Dilated proximal small bowel loops (arrow) secondary to obstuction by perforated diverticulitis

engorged vasa recta[18] and fluid. An abrupt zone of transition with normal bowel, presence of adjacent enlarged pericolonic lymph nodes, and colonic mural thickness greater than 1.5 cm suggest carcinoma. A follow-up scan following appropriate antibiotic therapy may sometimes be of benefit to distinguish diverticulitis from neoplasm. And in equivocal cases, histology can help differentiate.

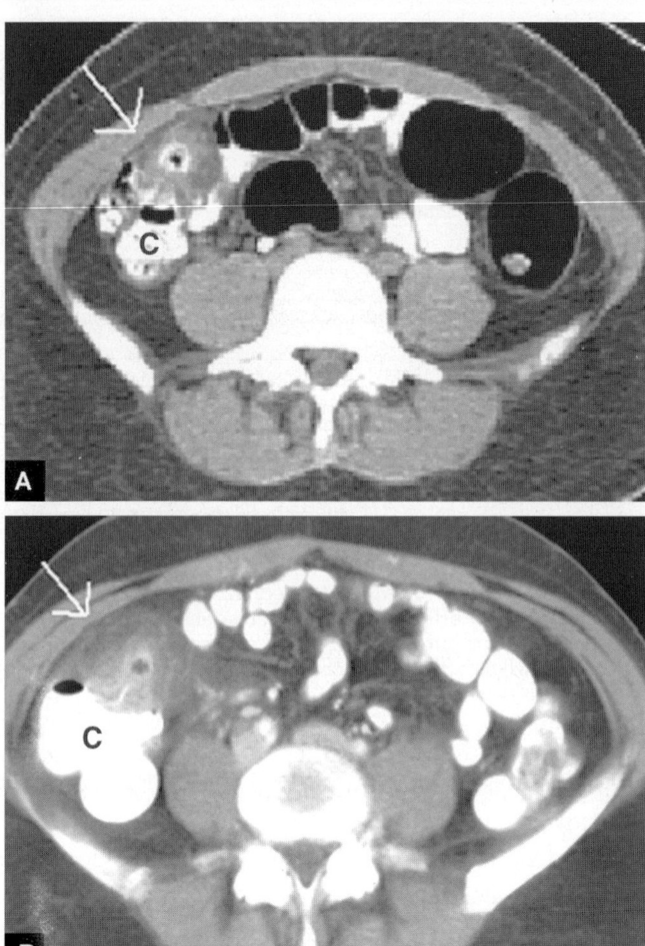

FIGURES 3.12A and B: Acute right lower quadrant pain. (A,B) Axial scans showing inflammed cecal diverticulum with eccentric cecal wall thickening and extensive mesenteric stranding (arrows) C= cecum

CT DIFFERENTIATING FEATURES OF DIVERTICULITIS AND COLON CARCINOMA[17-19] (Table 3.1)

TABLE 3.1

Feature	*Diverticulitis*	*Adenocarcinoma*
Length of the affected segment	Longer segment	Focal
Presence of diverticula	Almost always seen	May or may not be seen
Colonic wall thickening	Smooth eccentric	Irregular concentric with shouldering
Fat stranding	Disproportionate	Minimal or absent
Fluid	Present at mesenteric root	None
Lymphadenopathy	None	Present

ACUTE CHOLECYSTITIS

The clinical signs and symptoms of acute cholecystitis are nonspecific and in 62 to 85% of patients evaluated for clinically suspected cholecystitis, the symptoms may actually result from other causes.[20]

Though sonography has been the mainstay in evaluation of cholecystitis, CT scan as an initial technique in evaluation of the acute abdomen may be helpful. Also CT can readily detect complications of acute cholecystitis including perforation and gangrenous cholecystitis.

The CT features of acute cholecystitis are[21](Figure 3.13).

1. Mural thickening usually greater than 3 mm (distended gallbladder) in presence or absence of stones The sensitivity of CT for detection of stones is about 75%. Calcium containing stones are well seen. Cholesterol stones may be difficult to see. The use of narrow window settings may assist in the detection of gallstones on CT.
2. Enhancement of the inflamed gallbladder wall.
3. Pericholecystic stranding or fluid and blurring of the interface between the gallbladder and liver.
4. In addition, a transient increase in attenuation of the portion of the liver adjacent to the gallbladder has been reported in patients with acute cholecystitis.[22] This appearance has been attributed to result from hepatic artery hyperemia and early venous drainage (Figure 3.14).

Complications of cholecystitis include gangrenous cholecystitis and gallbladder rupture.

Gangrenous or emphysematous cholecystitis occurs commonly in diabetic patients usually due to infection by gas forming organisms.

CT is very sensitive and specific in diagnosing emphysematous cholecystitis. The CT findings include air in the gallbladder wall or lumen, intraluminal membranes, irregular or absent gallbladder wall, irregular gallbladder wall enhancement and pericholecystic abscess (Figure 3.15).

Diagnosis of emphysematous cholecystitis is important as it carries a mortality rate of up to 15%.[23]

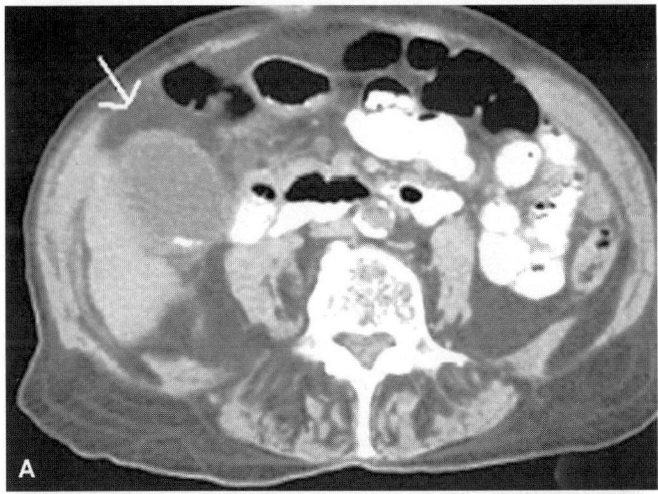

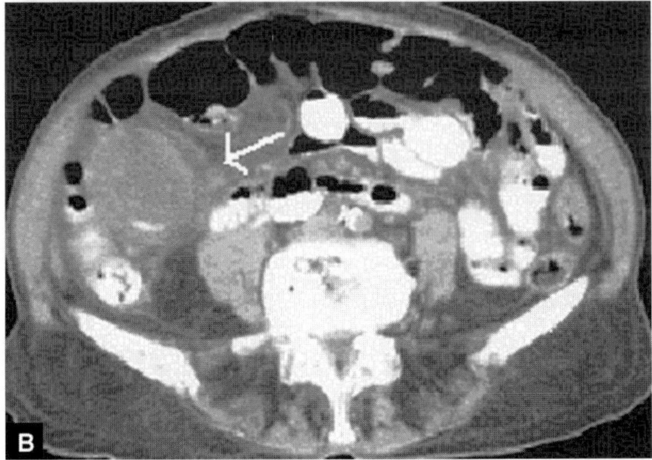

FIGURES 3.13A and B: Patient with acute right upper quadrant pain. (a) Axial nonintravenous contrast scan showing gall stones with thickened gallbladder wall (arrow) and hazy margins. (B) Scan showing thickened gallbladder wall and pericholecystic stranding (arrow) consistent with acute cholecystitis

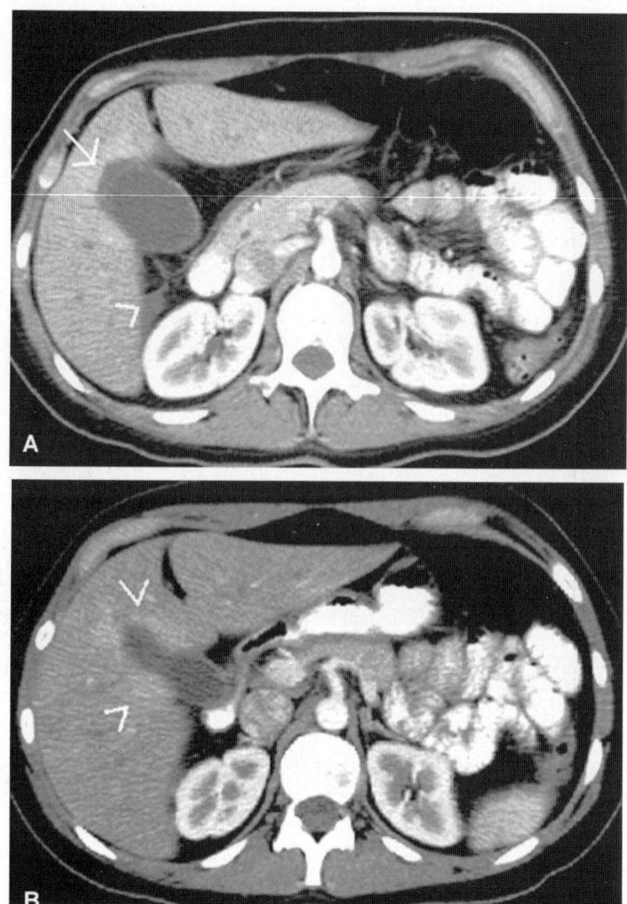

FIGURES 3.14A and B: Patient with suspected cholecystitis. (A) Axial scan with oral and intravenous contrast showing gallbladder wall edema (large arrow) and pericholecystic fluid (small arrow). (B) There is increased enhancement of the liver adjacent to the inflamed gallbladder (small arrows) due to hyperemia, a useful sign seen in acute cholecystitis on contrast scans

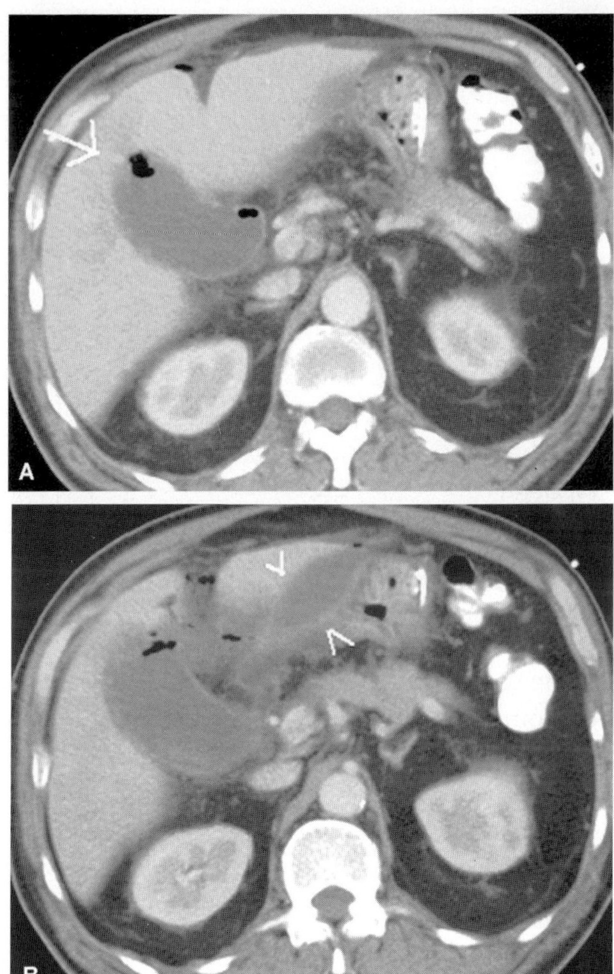

FIGURES 3.15A and B: Acute emphysematous cholecystitis with perforation. (A) Inflamed gallbladder with air within its lumen (large arrow). (B) Axial scan demonstrating perforated gallbladder with extensive stranding and intra-abdominal abscess (small arrows)

PANCREATITIS

Acute pancreatitis is an acute inflammatory condition of the pancreas that may extend to local and distant extrapancreatic tissues.

Causes of Acute Pancreatitis

- Gallstones—45%.
- Alcohol—35%.
- Others—10%.
- Medications.
- Hypercalcemia.
- Hypertriglyceridemia.
- Obstructive.
- Post ERCP.
- Hereditary.
- Viral.
- Vascular/ischemic.

Acute pancreatitis is generally classified into mild and severe forms. Mild pancreatitis also called interstitial or edematous pancreatitis is associated with minimal organ failure. It is usually self limiting without complication and followed by an uneventful recovery. On the other hand severe acute pancreatitis, also called necrotizing pancreatitis occurs in approximately 20% of patients and is associated with organ failure, high incidence of local complications including necrosis, infections, or pseudocyst formation.[24] Parenchymal pancreatic injury is the pathologic hallmark of this form of disease. The rationale for assessing the severity of acute pancreatitis is mainly from a practical standpoint. Mild-pancreatitis responds well to supportive therapy, whereas severe pancreatitis requires intensive monitoring and specific therapies and has a more severe outcome.

Imaging plays a vital role in the diagnosis of pancreatitis. An ideal imaging method is one that allows differentiation between patients with mild and those with severe pancreatitis, should be accurate, and easy to use.

Conventional abdominal radiographs while occasionally useful in detecting complication like pleural effusion, have no role in the early evaluation of disease severity.

Ultrasonography is useful in early pancreatitis to help evaluate for the presence of gallbladder or common duct stones. Ultrasound however has limited applications in early staging of the disease. Visualization of the pancreas is often impaired by overlying bowel gas and the detection of intraparenchymal and retroperitoneal fluid collections in the setting of pancreatic necrosis is typically poor.

Helical CT plays a vital role in the diagnosis and clinical management. CT is used to stage the severity and has greatly improved the clinical outcome. CT can detect signs of early pancreatitis, detect pancreatic necrosis, assess for extrapancreatic complications, and help differentiate mild from severe pancreatitis.

CT FEATURES OF PANCREATITIS

The early CT findings of acute pancreatitis reflect edema of the gland and the surrounding fat may be normal in up to 28% of mild cases.[25] The entire gland may become enlarged and edematous with a shaggy irregular contour (Figure 3.16). The surrounding peripancreatic fat shows high attenuation, the vascular margins are cuffed and the fascial planes are thickened. Focal pancreatitis occurs in 10 to 18% of patients and is usually associated with stone disease.[26]

In more advanced cases, intraglandular extravasation of pancreatic fluid leads to formation of small intrapancreatic fluid collections. In necrotizing pancreatitis, the gland becomes enlarged and is surrounded by high attenuation exudates. Necrotic parenchyma shows decreased or no enhancement and is sharply-demarcated from the normally-enhancing viable tissue (Figures 3.17A and B). The body and the tail are usually involved, however the head is often spared because of its rich collateral vascular network. The peripancreatic fluid collections dissect and penetrate through the fascial planes. These collections typically accumulate in the lesser sac, anterior pararenal space and anterior interfascial space. CT is also useful in revealing vascular complications such as pseudoaneurysms and splenic and portal vein thrombosis.

CT can help predict patient outcome by delineating necrosis. Also the CT severity index introduced in 1994 by Balthazar and colleagues was a significant advancement in the assessment of patients with acute pancreatitis.[27,28] This CT severity index, which is based on scoring the presence and degree of pancreatic inflammation and pancreatic necrosis, not only allows accurate differentiation of mild from severe pancreatitis but also numerically correlates with the patients prognosis (Table 3.2).

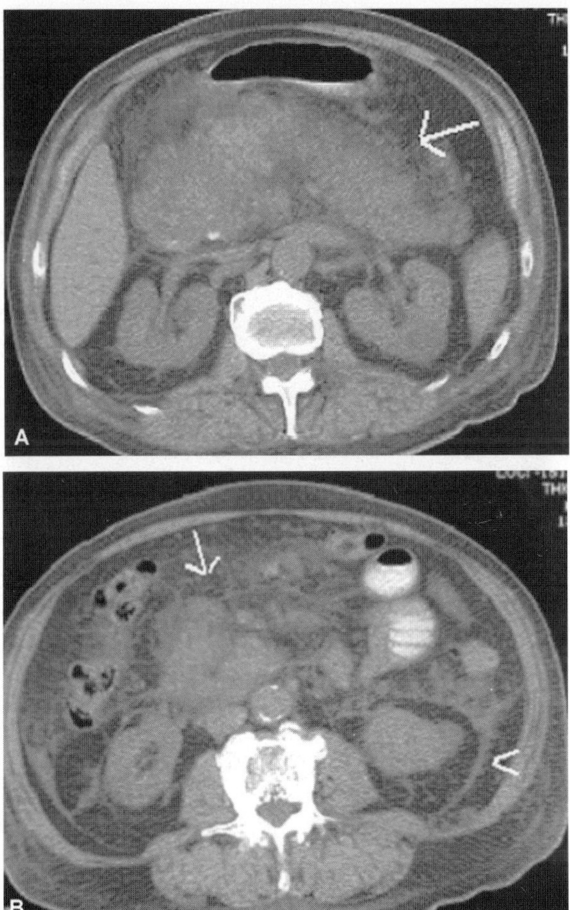

FIGURES 3.16A and B: Acute abdominal pain and clinical suspicion of acute pancreatitis. (a) Axial non-contrast scan showing enlarged and edematous pancreas with peripancreatic stranding (arrow). (B) caudal scan showing peripancreatic stranding (large arrow) and thickening of para-renal fascia (small arrow) consistent with acute pancreatitis

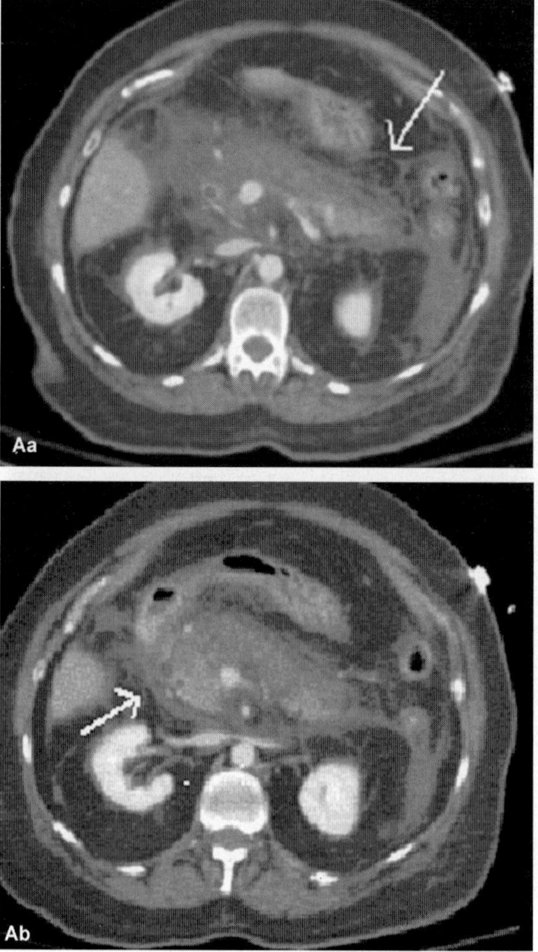

FIGURE 3.17A: Patient with severe mid-abdominal pain and suspected pancreatitis (a,b) axial scans with intravenous contrast demonstrating extensive peripancreatic inflammation and fluid,the pancreas appears hypodense with no enhancement, except for a small portion of the head (arrow in figure b), consistent with necrotic pancreatitis

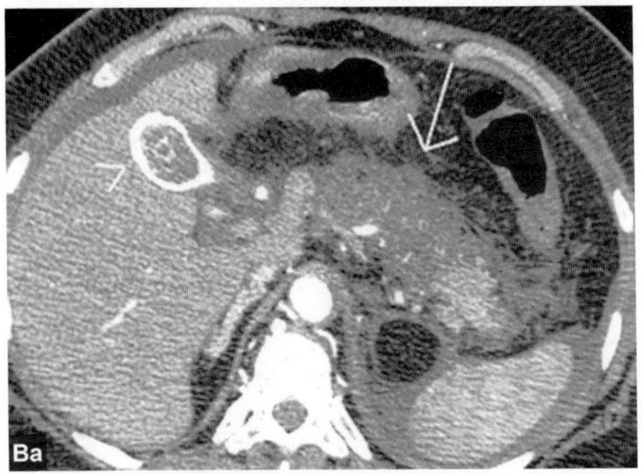

3.17Ba

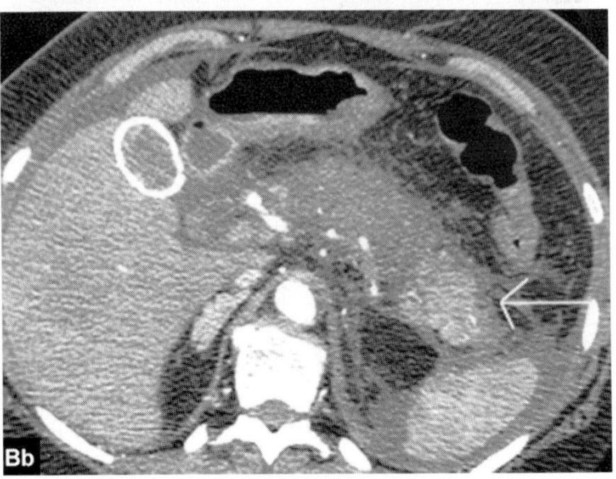

3.17Bb

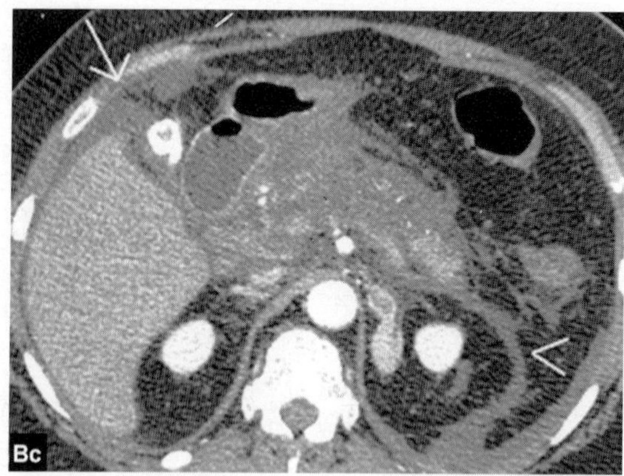

3.17Bc

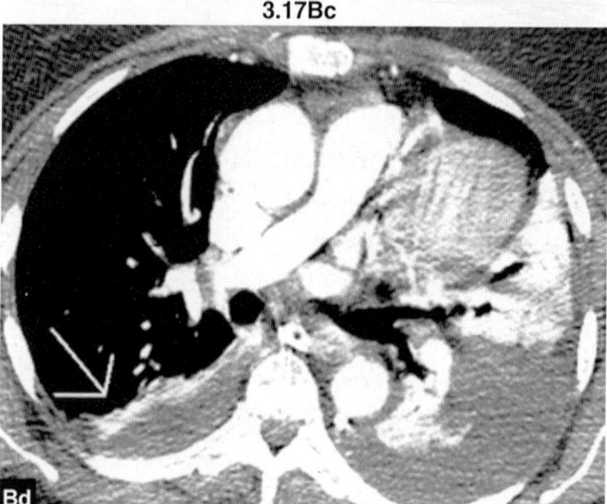

3.17Bd

FIGURE 3.17B: Patient presented with severe upper abdominal pain and suspected pancreatitis. (a,b) Axial scans with intravenous contrast demonstrating an inflamed pancreas, the pancreas appears hypodense with no enhancement, except for a small portion of the tail (large arrow in figure b),incidentally noted is porcelain gallbladder with gall stones (small arrow in figure a). (c) Caudal scan showing severe peripancreatic stranding and free fluid (arrows). (d) Scan at the lung bases showing bilateral pleural effusions (arrows)

TABLE 3.2: CT severity index

Prognostic Indicator	*Points*
Pancreatic inflammation.	0
Normal pancreas.	1
Focal or diffuse enlargement of the pancreas.	2
Intrinsic pancreatic abnormalities with inflammatory changes in peripancreatic fat.	3
Single ill-defined fluid collection or phlegmon.	4
Two or more fluid collections or presence of gas in or adjacent to the pancreas.	5
Pancreatic necrosis	
None	0
< 30%	2
> 30-50%	4
>50%	6

A modified CT severity index for acute pancreatitis has been reported in the literature.[29] This index is a modification of the previous CT severity index and takes into consideration other features like extrapancreatic findings such as pleural fluid, ascites, vascular complications, and involvement of the gastrointestinal tract. It has been shown to correlate more closely with patient outcome especially with the length of the hospital stay and the development of organ failure (Table 3.3).

CT IN EVALUATION OF RENAL COLIC

Renal colic is a common cause of acute abdomen. The usual underlying pathologies include renal stones, ureteral obstruction, and acute pyelonephritis.

Table 3.3: Modified CT severity index

Prognostic Indicator	*Points*
Pancreatic Inflammation Normal	0
Intrinsic pancreatic abnormalities with or without inflammatory changes in peripancreatic fat.	2
Pancreatic or peripancreatic fluid collection or peripancreatic necrosis.	4
Pancreatic necrosis.	
None	0
<30%	2
>30%	4
Extrapancreatic complications (one or more of pleural effusion, ascites, vascular complications, Parenchymal complications or gastrointestinal tract involvement.	

The clinical manifestations are acute flank pain on either side, hematuria or symptoms relating to micturition.

Although plain radiography has been the initial mode of evaluation, the diagnosis is frequently uncertain despite obtaining plain films.

Further the exact location of the calculus often remains unclear, the degree of ureteral obstruction cannot be determined and other conditions presenting as flank pain cannot be excluded.

Sonography hass proven excellent in detecting renal and upper/lower ureteric calculi. However, it is operator dependent, may be obscured by bowel gas and cannot always exclude other conditions presenting as flank pain.

Unenhanced Helical CT has become the imaging technique of choice in patients with acute flank pain in whom diagnosis is uncertain. All kinds of stones are visible on CT, with the exception of crystal deposits of protease inhibitor Indinavir used in HIV treatment.[30] In addition to identifying stones in the ureter, CT can also detect secondary signs of ureteral obstruction and also differentiate between ureteric calculi or phleboliths.[31] CT is fast, accurate and can evaluate associated conditions mimicking ureterolithiasis.

CT TECHNIQUE

The CT examinations for suspected ureterolithiasis are performed without IV or oral contrast. A narrow collimation of 5 mm is recommended to detect small ureteric calculi. Scans are covered from the level of diaphragm to the symphysis pubis. Multiplanar reconstructions may or may not be necessary.

CT APPROACH TO URETERAL OBSTRUCTION

Interpretation should begin with inspection for secondary signs of ureteral obstruction.

The secondary signs of obstruction are (Figures 3.18 to 3.20):[32]

1. Asymmetric perinephric, periureteral fat stranding.
2. Dilatation of intrarenal collection system and hydroureter.
3. Unilateral renal enlargement
4. A helpful secondary sign is the unilateral absence of white pyramids (Figure 3.21).[33]

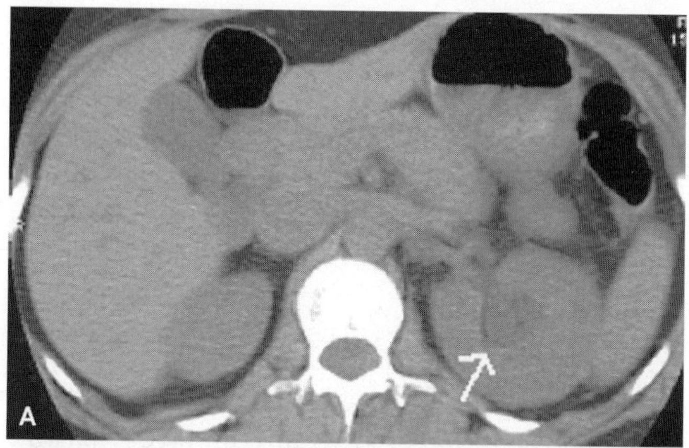

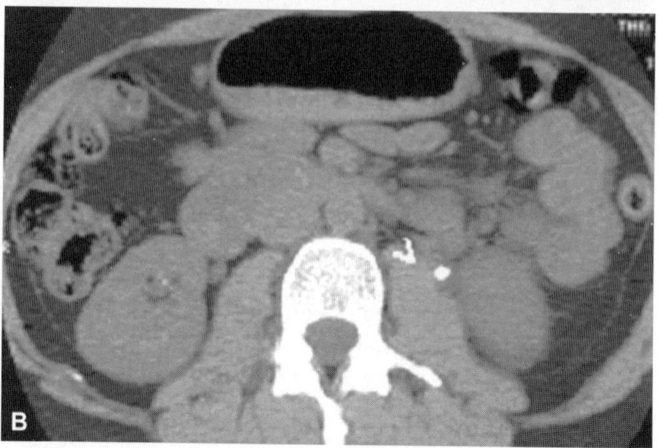

FIGURES 3.18A and B: Patient with acute left flank pain and suspected renal stones. (A) Non-contrast CT showing fullness of the left renal calyces (arrow). (B) Caudal section showing the calculus in the left proximal ureter small (arrow)

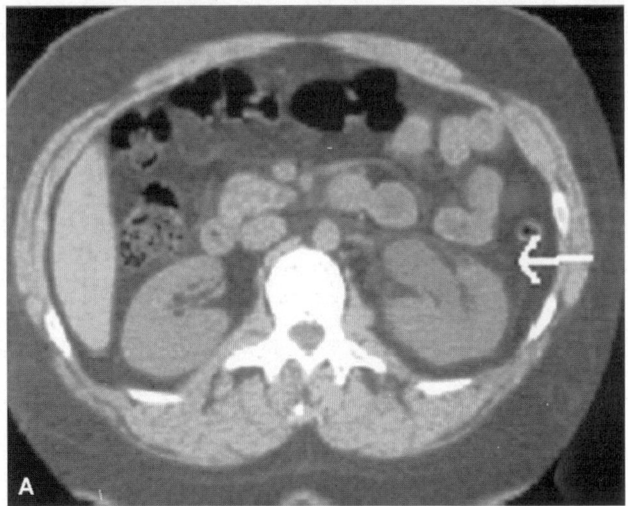

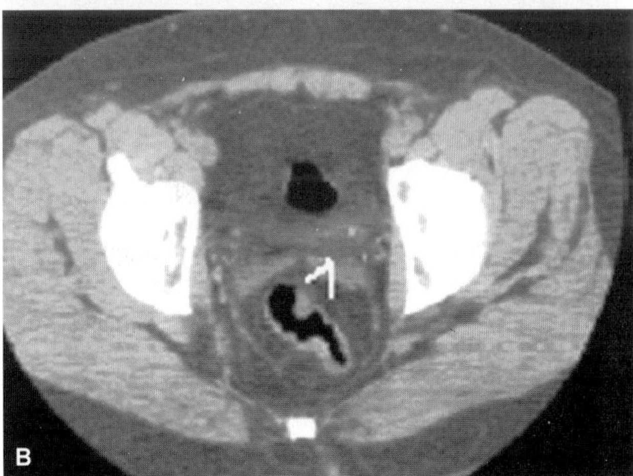

FIGURES 3.19A and B: Patient with acute left flank pain and hematuria. (A) Noncontrast scan showing left-sided hydronephrosis (arrow). (B) A small calcific density is seen at the left ureterovesical junction (small arrow) consistent with a ureterovesical junction calculus

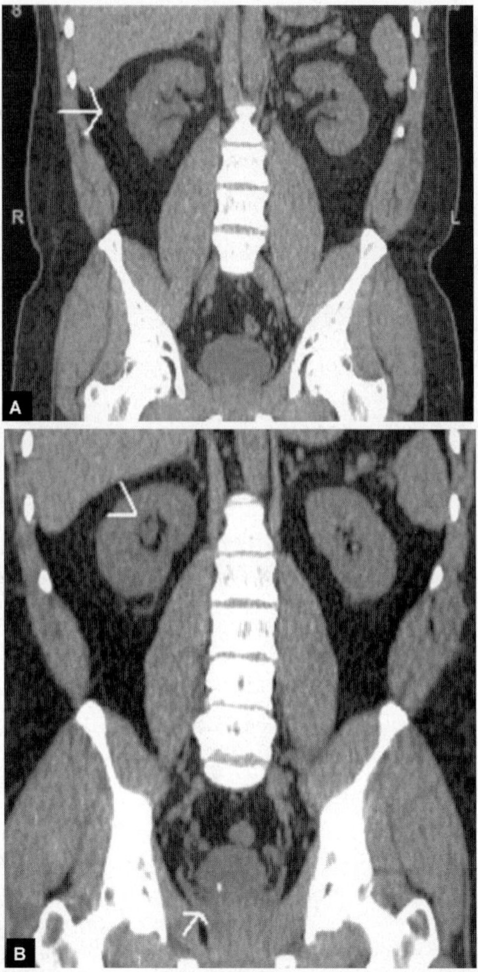

FIGURES 3.20A and B: Coronal reformats add additional benefit in evaluating renal colic. (a) Non-contrast coronal reformat showing mild right hydronephrosis (large arrow). (b) Coronal reformat showing fullness of the right renal pelvis (small arrow) and right ureterovesical junction calculus (large arrow)

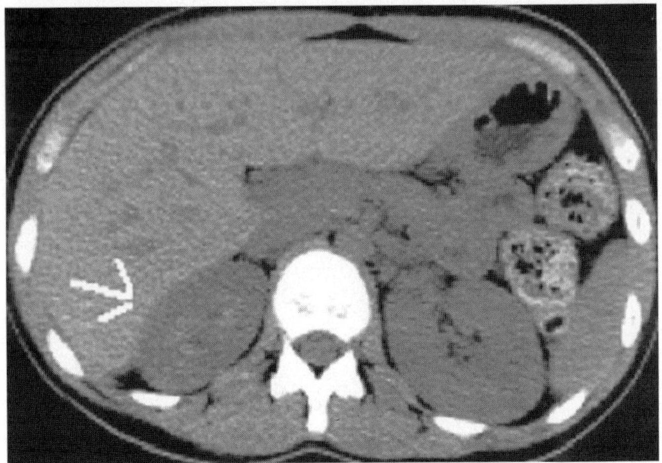

FIGURE 3.21: 'The white pyramid signs. The white pyramid sign represent high attenuation renal pyramids (arrow) seen in the kidneys incidentally on non-contrast CT. Note—there is absence of white pyramid on the left side indicating tubular hydronephrosis, an early sign of obstruction

1. Bilateral perinephric stranding is a common nonspecific finding on CT in older patients. This usually results from fluid collection within the septa of perinephric fat due to increased lymphatic pressure.

   Unilateral or asymmetric perinephric stranding is abnormal. It is indicative of obstruction or pyelonephritis. Also sometimes definite perinephric fluid is noted. This is suggestive of extravasated urine as a result of forniceal rupture (Figure 3.22A).

   Subtle perinephric stranding is difficult to visualize. Look at the upper or lower poles and compare with the contralateral kidney.

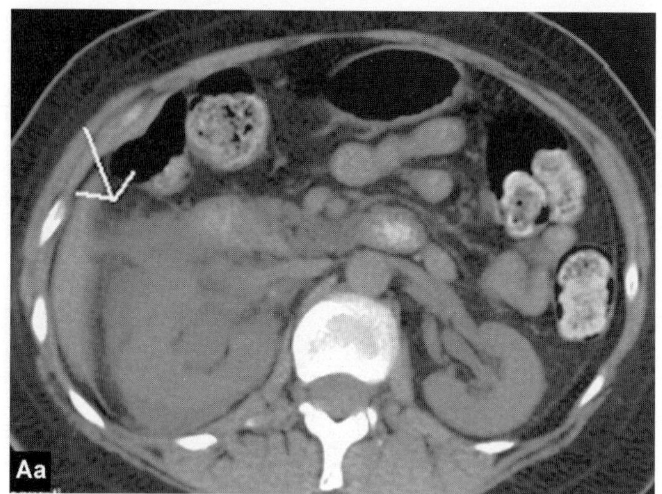

3.22Aa

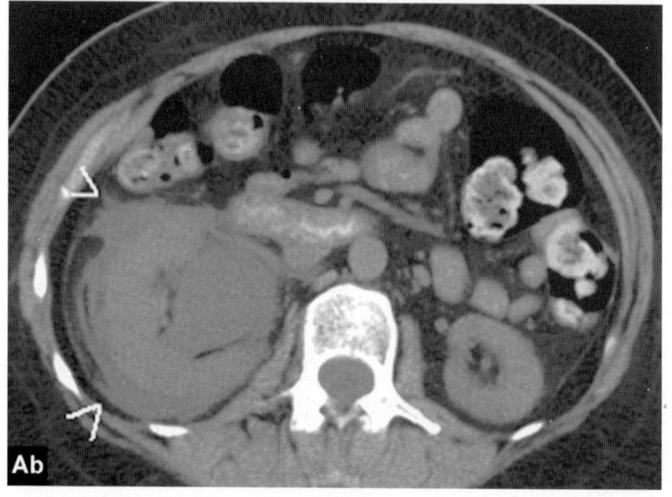

3.22Ab

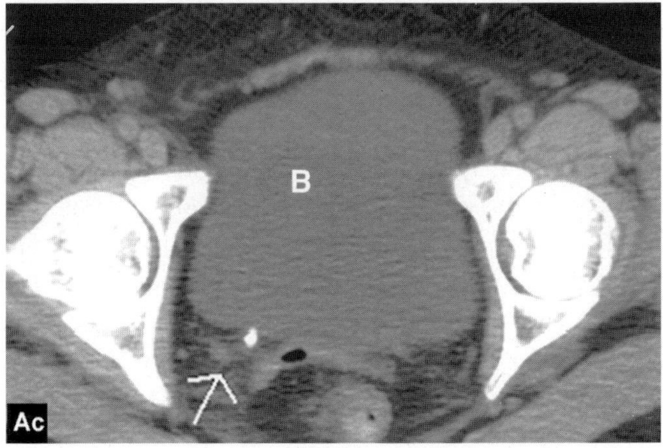

3.22Ac

FIGURE 3.22A: Patient with acute right flank pain and hematuria. (a) noncontrast scan showing moderate right sided hydronephrosis and extensive perinephric stranding (arrow). (b) There is moderate hydronephrosis with perinephric fluid (small arrows) suggestive of forniceal rupture. (c) axial scan at the level of bladder showing a terminal ureteric calculus (arrow)

2. Next evaluate for collecting system dilatation.

   Always look at the upper or lower pole calyces. Extrarenal pelvis may lead to apparent dilation of central renal collecting system. Also small peripelvic cysts mimick hydronephrosis on noncontrast CT. Dilated calyces appear as rounded fluid filled structures and obliterate the renal fat.

   When there is ureteral dilation, trace the ureter from renal pelvis to the bladder. A thrombosed gonadal vein may mimic a dilated ureter.
3. Unilateral renal enlargement. T intrarenal pressure results in mild anlargement and altered shape of the

kidney which is again a subtle sign of early hydronephrosis. However, renal enlargement may also be seen in acute pyelonephritis.

4. Another useful sign is the unilateral absence of white pyramid. Bilateral high attenuation renal pyramids are seen in the kidney incidentally on non-contrast CT. The absence of white pyramids indicates tubular hydronephrosis, decreasing attenuation of the medullary pyramids on the obstructed side.

IDENTIFYING URETERAL CALCULI

After evaluation of secondary signs look for calcifications within the ureter. The entire course of the ureter has to be followed. CT can detect stones as small as 2 mm. The common difficulty is differentiating distal ureteral stones from phleboliths, although calcification within the ureter excludes phleboliths. However, it is not always easy to differentiate the two in the absence of ureteral dilation. A helpful sign is the soft tissue "rim sign" (Figure 3.22B). Most of the ureteral stones are surrounded by a rim of soft tissue because of edema of the ureteral wall where as phleboliths are surrounded by fat.[34]

Stones at the level of the ureterovesical junction may be sometimes difficult to differentiate from a calculus that has recently passed from the ureter into the bladder. Rescanning the patient in the prone position may help differentiate recently passed stones that fall anteriorly into the dependent portion of the urinary bladder, whereas stones impacted at the ureterovescical junction do not.[35]

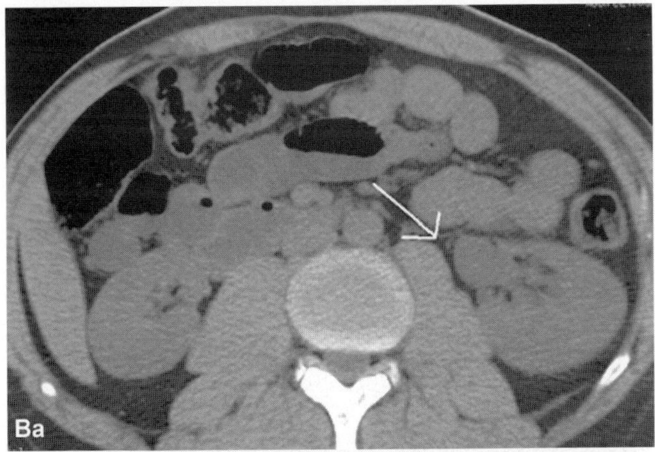

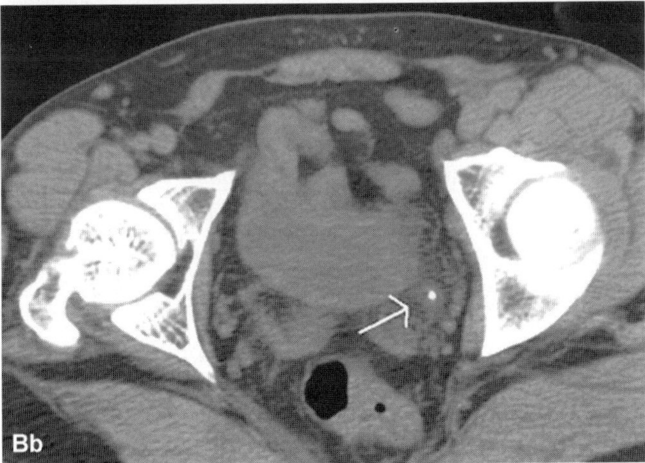

FIGURE 3.22B: Patient with acute left flank pain radiating to groin. (a) Noncontrast axial scan showing left hydronephrosis (arrow). (b) Scan at the level of the pelvis demonstrating a terminal ureteric calculus with the 'rim sign' (arrow).The rim sign helps in differentiating distal ureteral stones from phleboliths. Most of the ureteral stones are surrounded by a rim of soft tissue whereas phleboliths are surrounded by fat

Finally when no ureteral stone is detected, but secondary signs of obstruction are present, the scans are interpreted as positive. The differential diagnosis includes a recently passed stone, pyelonephritis or urinary tract obstruction unrelated to stones. Further evaluation with contrast CT is recommended.

POINTS TO REMEMBER

1. Look for secondary signs of obstruction like asymmetric perinephric stranding, unilateral absence of white pyramids.
2. Always look at the upper or lower pole calyces for early calyceal dilation
3. Soft tissue rim sign may differentiate ureteral stones from phleboliths.
4. Prone scan may help differentiate recently passed stones from ureterovesical calculus.

PEPTIC ULCER DISEASES AND GASTROINTESTINAL PERFORATIONS

Patients with peptic ulcer disease often present with acute abdomen with no localizing signs and symptoms. Clinically it may be indistinguishable from acute pancreatitis or cholecystitis. Helical CT is normally the first investigation recommended in acute abdomen.

The CT finding of peptic ulcer disease includes focal mural thickening of the antrum or duodenum (Figure 3.23). These may also be also accompanied by inflam-

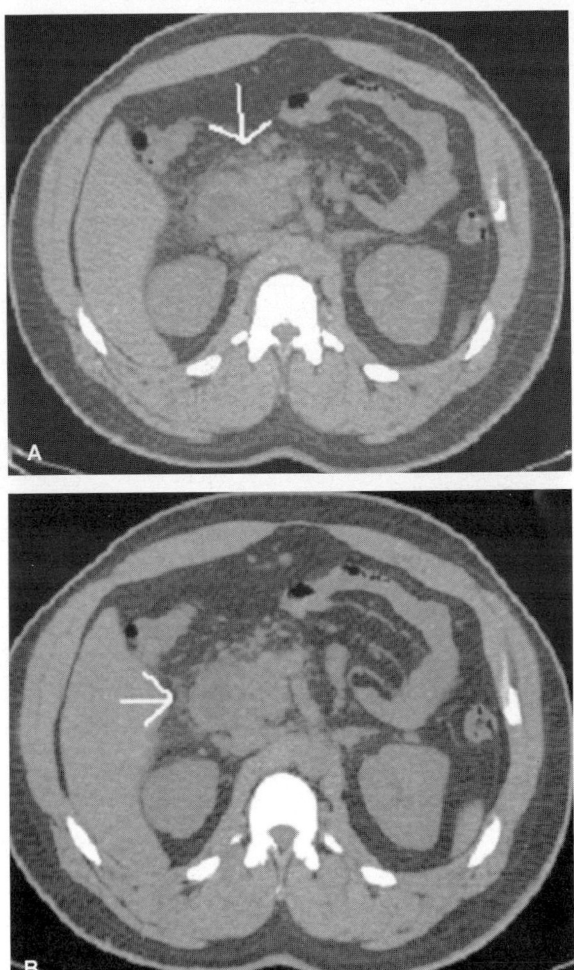

FIGURES 3.23A and B: Patient with acute upper abdominal pain with suspicion of cholecystitis. (A,B) Axial non-contrast scans showing thickening of the duodenum with adjacent periduodenal fat stranding suggestive of duodenitis

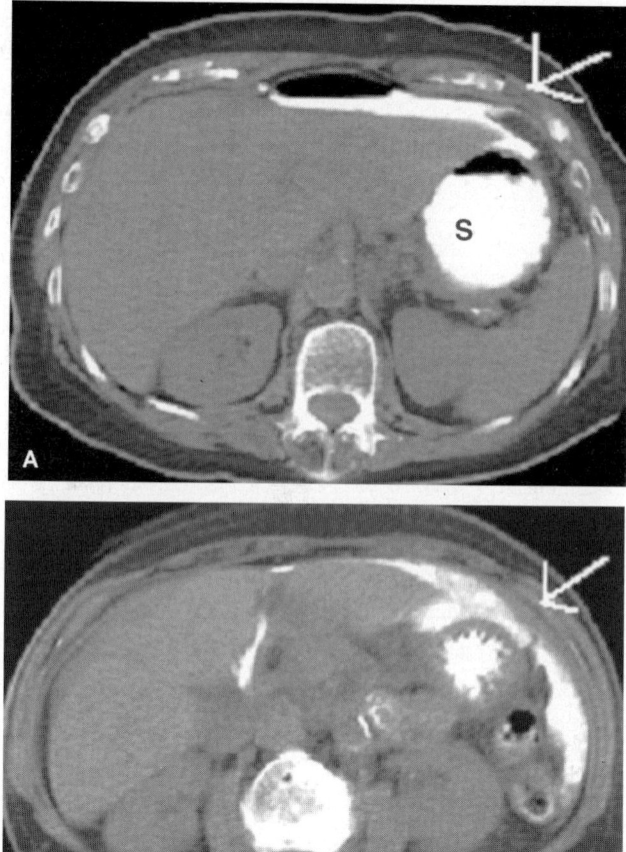

FIGURES 3.24A and B: An example of perforated gastric ulcer. (A,B) Axial scans with oral contrast demonstrating extravasation of oral contrast (arrows) in the peritoneum consistent with perforated gastric ulcer S=stomach

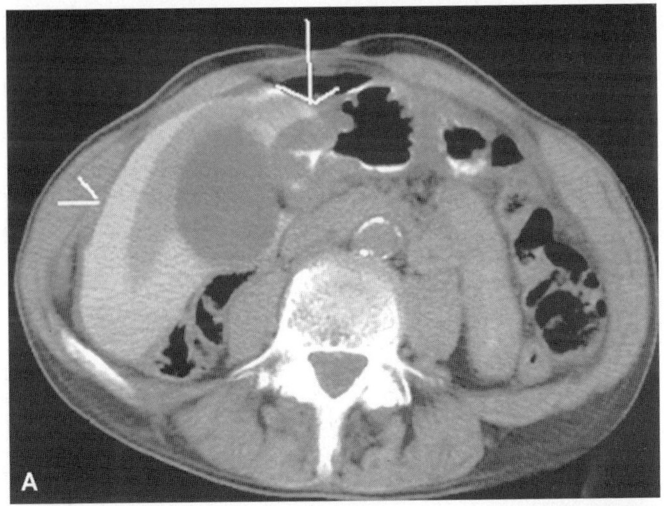

3.25A

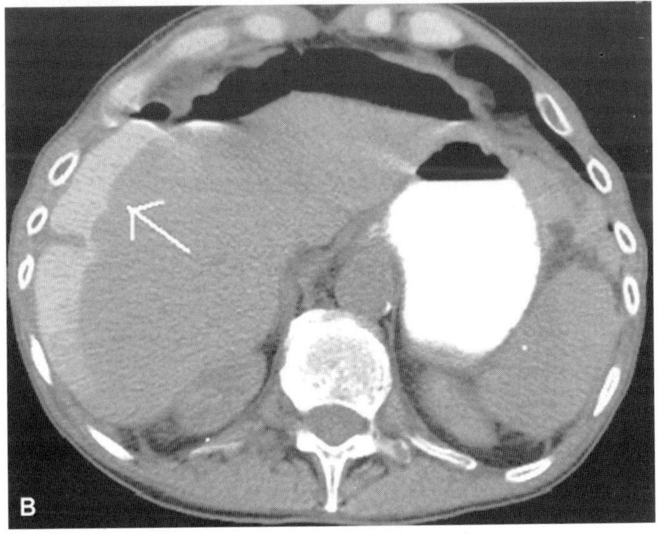

3.25B

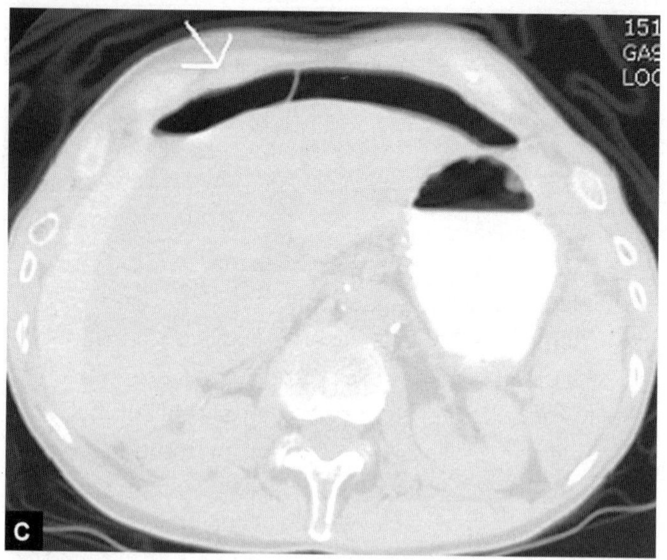

3.25C

FIGURES 3.25A to C: Patient with history of peptic diseases presenting with severe upper abdominal pain. (a) Axial scan with oral contrast showing thickened distal stomach (large arrow). (b) Same scan demonstrating extravasation of oral contrast (large arrow). (C) Scan in lung window setting showing free intraperitoneal air consistent with perforated peptic ulcer

matory changes in the adjacent mesentery. Occasionally an active ulcer or perforation is identified.[36, 37] CT may demonstrate free air and extravasation of oral contrast in the case of a perforated ulcer (Figure 3.24).

Gastrointestinal perforation indicates catastrophic complications of many acute intra-abdominal pathologic like peptic ulcer disease, diverticulitis, ischemic bowel disease, closed loop obstruction, and many other conditions.

Helical CT is the investigation of choice for evaluating patients with gastrointestinal perforation. CT can detect pneumoperitoneum or signs of peritonitis, which often may be misdiagnosed as other acute conditions.

Helical CT can also detect the site of perforation (Figure 3.25). Administration of oral and IV contrast may greatly assist in the identification of the site of perforation. Loculated fluid and gas, focal mesenteric stranding or focal enhancement of the parietal peritoneum can help pinpoint the site of perforation. Occasionally, in case of a large perforation, the site of extravasation of oral contrast may be visualized, indicating the site of perforation

REFERENCES

1. Balthazar EJ, Rofsky NM, and Zucker R. Appendicitis the impact of computed tomography imaging on negative appendectomy and perforation rates. AMJ Gastroentered 1998; 93:768-71.
2. Anderson RE, Hugander A, Thulin AJG. Diagnostic accuracy and perforation rate in appendicitis; association with age and sex of patient and with appendectomy rate. Eur J Surgery 1992; 15:37-41.
3. Balthazar EJ, Meigbow. AJ, Siegel SE, Birnbaum BA. Appendicitis: Prospective evaluation with high resolution CT, Radiology 1991; 180:21-4.
4. Picken G, Ellis H, Dixon AK. The normal vermiform appendix of computed tomography. Visualization and anatomical location. Clin Anat 1993; 6:9-14.
5. Weltman DI, Yu J, Kru meancker J, Huang S, Moh P. Dagnosis of acute appendicitis; Comparison of 5 and 10 mm CT section in the same patient. Radiology 2000; 216: 172-177.

6. Rao PM, Technical and interpretative pit falls of appendiceal CT imaging. AJR 1998; 171:419-25.
7. Rao PM, Rhea JT, Novelline RA, Mostafavi AA, McCabe CJ, Lawrason JN, Berger DL, et al. Helical CT technique for the diagnosis of appendicitis; prospective evaluation of a focused appendix CT examination. Radiology 1997; 202: 139-44.
8. Lane MJ, Katz Ds, Ross BA. Clatice-Eangle TL, Mindelzun RE, Jeffrey RB Jr. Unenhanced helical CT for suspected acute appendicitis.
9. Rao PM, Rhea JT, Novelline RA, Mostafavi AA, Lawrason JN, McCabe CJ. Helical CT combined with contrast material administered only through the colon for imaging of suspected appendicitis AJR AM JR Roentgenal 1997; 169: 1275-80.
10. Rao PM, Wittenberg J, McDowell RK, Rhea JT, Novelline RA. Appendicitis; use of arrowhead sing for diagnosis at CT Radiology 1997-202:303-66.
11. Rao PM, Rhea JT, Novelline RA. Distal appendicitis, CT appearance and diagnosis. Radiology 1997;204: 704-12.
12. Lane MJ, Katx DS, Liu Dm, Wolanske KA, Mindelzun Re, Jeffrey RB Jr. Establishing an alternative diagnosis on unenhanced helical CT for acute appendicitis; experience with 237 consecutive patient scans (abst). Radiology 1998; 209; 368.
13. Rao PM, Boland GW, Imaging of acute right lower abdominal quadrant pain. Clinical Radiology 1998; 53: 639-49.
14. Ming S-C, Diverticular disease of the colon. In Ming S-C, Gold man H (Eds): Pathology of the gastrointenstial tract, 2nd ed. Battimore; William and Wilkins, 1999: 801-18
15. Wescner SD, Dailey TH. The initial management of the left lower quadrant peritonitis, Discolon Rectum 1986; 29: 635-8.
16. Johnson CD, Baker ME, Rice RP et al. Diagnosis of acute colonic diverticulitis. Comparison of barium enema and CT. AJR 1987; 148: 541-6.

17. Padidar AM, Jeffrey RJ Jr, Midelzun RE, Dolph JF, Differentiating sigmoid diverticulitis from carcinoma on CT scan; mesenteric inflammation suggests diverticulitis; AJR 1994; 163: 81-3.
18. Chintapalli K.N, Chopra S, Ghiatas AA, Esola CC Fields SF, Dodd GD 3rd Diverticulitis versus colon cancer; differentiation with helical CT findings, Radiology 1999; 210: 429-35.
19. Jang HJ, Lim HK, Lee WJ, Kim Ey, Kim SH, Acute diverticulitis of the cecum and ascending; the value of thin sectional helical CT findings in excluding colonic carcinoma. AJR AMJ Roentgenol 2000; 174: 1397-1402.
20. Paulson EK Acute cholecystitis. CT findings semin ultrasound CT MR 2000; 21: 56-63.
21. Fidler, Joint Paulson EK, Layfield L CT evaluation of acute cholecystitis; findings and usefulness in diagnosis. AJR 1996; 166: 1085-88.
22. Yamashita K Jin MJ, Hirose Y, et al CT findings of transient focal increased attenuation of the liver adjacent to the gall bladder in acute cholecystitis; AJR 1995; 164: 343-6.
23. Gray son DE, Abott RM, Levy AD, et al. Emphysematous infections of the abdomen and pelvis; a pictorial review. Radio Graphics 2002; 22: 543-61.
24. Bradley EL 111. A clinically-based classification system for acute pancreatitis; summary of the international symposium on Acute Pancreatitis. Atlanta GA, September II through 13, 1992. Arch Surg 1993; 128: 586-90.
25. Baron TH, Morgan DE, Acute necrotising pancreatitis. N Engl J Med 1999; 340 1412-17.
26. Yassa NA, Agostini JT, Ralls PW, Accuracy of CT in estimating the extent of pancreatic necrosis. Clin Radiol 1997; 21: 407-10.
27. Bathazar EJ, Robinson DL, Megibow AJ, Ranson JHC. Acute pancreatitis; value of CT in establishing prognosis Radiology 1990; 174: 331-6.
28. Balthazar EJ, Freeny PC, Vansonnenberg E. Imaging and intervention in acute pancreatitis. Radiology 1994; 193: 297-306.

29. Koenraad J, Mortele, Walter Wiesner, Lisa Intriere, Shridhar shankar, Kelly H Zoee. A modified CT severity index for evaluating acute pancreatitis. AJR 2004; 183: 1261-5.
30. Blake SP, Mc Nicholas MMJ, Raptopoulas V. Nonopaque crystal deposition causing ureteric obstruction in patients with HIV undergoing indinavir therapy. AJR AMJ Roentgenol 1998; 171:717-20.
31. Traubici Jt, Neithlich JD, Smith RC, Distinguishing pelvic phleboliths from distal ureteral stones on unenhanced helical CT; is there a radiolucent center ? AJR Am Joint Roentgenol 1999; 172: 13-7.
32. Smith R C, Verga M. Dalrymple N, Mc Carthy S, Rosenfield AT. Acute ureteral obstruction ; Value of secondary signs on helical unenhanced CT. AJR Am Joint Roentgenol 1996; 167: 1109-13.
33. Roychowdhary A, Makris J, Colby J M, et al. Unilateral absence of the 'white pyramid' sign on noncontrast CT; a sign of tubular hydronephrosis? Presented at the 98th Meeting of the American Roentgen Ray Society, Scientific Session 33, Streaky atelectasis is noted Francisco, Calif, April 26-May 1, 1998.
34. Heneghan JH, Dalrymple NC, Verga M, Rosenfield AT. Smith RC Soft tissue 'rim' sign in the diagnosis of ureteral calculi with use of unenhanced helical. CT Radiology 1997; 202: 709-11.
35. Levine J. Neitlich J, Smith RC, The value of prone scanning to distinguish ureterovesical junction stones from ureteral stones that have passed into the bladder; leave no stone unturned. AJR AmJ Roentgenol 1999; 172: 977-81.
36. Madrazo BL, Halpert RD, Sandler MA, Pearlberg JL. Computed tomographic findings in penetrating peptic ulcer. Radiology 1984; 153: 751-4.
37. Jacobs JM, Hill MC, Steinberg WM, peptic ulcer disease. CT evaluation. Radiology 1991; 178: 745-8

CT IN CHOLEDOCHOLITHIASIS

Choledocholithiasis[1] is seen in approximately 6–12% of patients undergoing cholecystectomy. Common bile duct stones may be asymptomatic but can often lead to biliary colic, cholangitis, jaundice, or pancreatitis.

In patients in whom choledocholithiasis is clinically suspected, transabdominal sonography is the most commonly used initial examination to screen for gallbladder disease because of its low cost and relatively high accuracy. However, in patients with symptoms that are not specific, such as abdominal pain, or with symptoms that are suspicious for pancreaticocholedochal disease, helical CT performed with IV contrast material is widely used for the initial evaluation. Consequently, radiologists need to recognize the imaging findings of common bile duct stones on contrast-enhanced CT scans because that is often the first opportunity they have to diagnose a common bile duct stone. Although ERCP, MRCP, and endoscopic sonography are more sensitive than CT, these modalities are usually not the first imaging tests performed for evaluating common bile duct stones.

CT PROTOCOLS[2]

(A) NONCONTRAST ENHANCED HELICAL CT

CT without oral or intravenous contrast is less sensitive than CT cholangiogram, but is better than oral and IV contrast enhanced CT.

No oral contrast (why?)→refluxed oral contrast material may obscure the stones and make recognition more difficult.

No intravenous contrast (why?)→Distinguishing enhancing bile duct mucosa from common bile duct stones can be challenging and result in both decreased sensitivity and specificity of contrast-enhanced helical CT (especially in the setting of cholangitis due to associated infection or in patients with AIDS cholangitis).

(B) CT WITH ORAL AND INTRAVENOUS CONTRAST

MOST widely used modality for investigating vague abdominal complaints , where choledocholithiasis/ biliary dilatation are diagnosed incidentally (therefore it is important that the radiologists should be able to recognize the imaging findings of common bile duct stones on contrast-enhanced CT scans and be aware of the associated pitfalls)

(C) HCT CHOLANGIOGRAPHY

After the initial emergency imaging evaluation, CT may be performed specifically to look for choledocholithiasis. Helical CT is performed following opacification of biliary tract with oral cholangiographic contrast agents (ipanoic acid) or an intravenous infusion of a cholangiographic contrast material(meglumine salt of adipiodone). The patient is also given about 500 ml water orally to distend the stomach and duodenum. (sensitivity 85%, specificity 88%, and accuracy 86%) Limitations: not helpful in the acute setting, contraindicated in jaundiced patients.

Appropriate CT technique for the purpose of detection of choledocholithiasis:

- Thin collimation of 2.5–5.0 mm
- Overlapping reconstructed axial CT scans obtained at 2-mm increments
- Highest kilovoltage setting(to increase the chances of distinguishing these stones from bile—because most stones are composed primarily of cholesterol , resulting in an attenuation similar to that of bile)

Appropriate viewing:

- Bile window settings (i.e. adjusting the window level setting to the mean attenuation of the common bile duct and the window width to 150 H)
- Multiplanar reformatted oblique coronal images through the common bile duct
- Magnifying the scans
- Using cine mode or scrolling through CT scans on a PACS workstation

CT FEATURES OF CHOLEDOCHOLITHIASIS[4]

Types of stones as seen on CT[3]:

A. Calcified
B. Soft tissue density
C. Low density

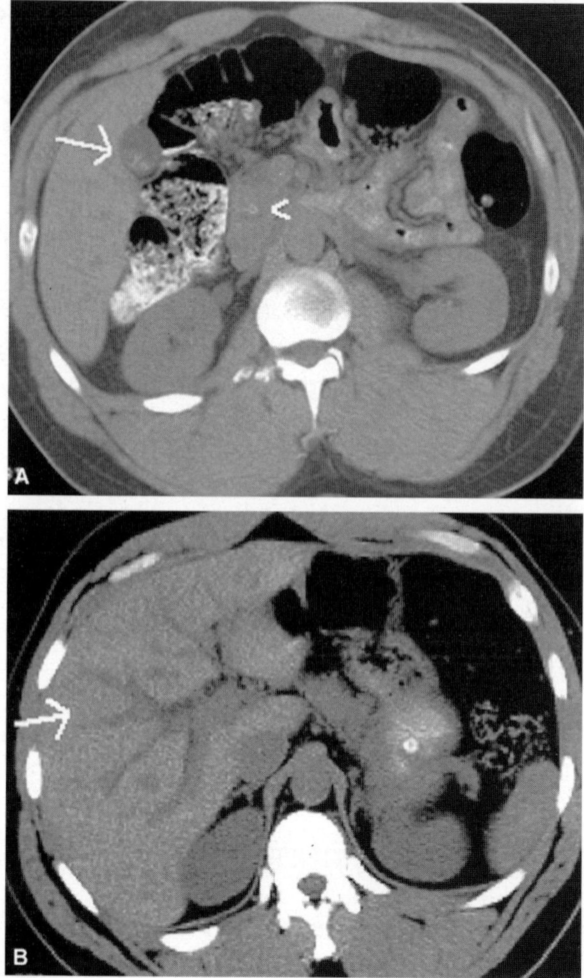

FIGURES 3.26A and B: Acute right upper quadrant pain. (A) Non-contrast scan showing multiple gall bladder stones (large arrow) with a calcified stone in the common bile duct (small arrow). (B) Superior scan showing dilated intrahepatic bile ducts

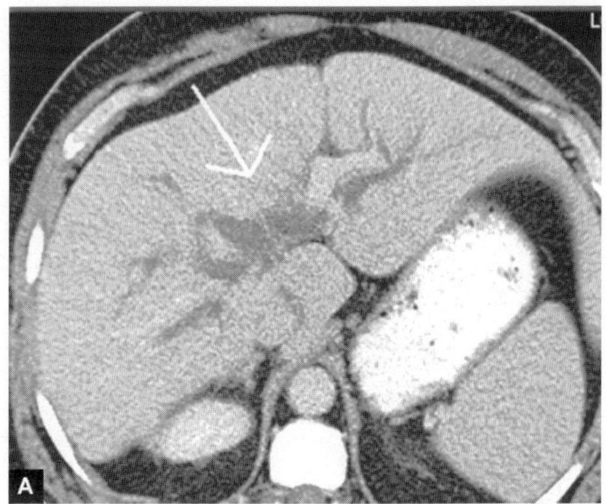

3.27A

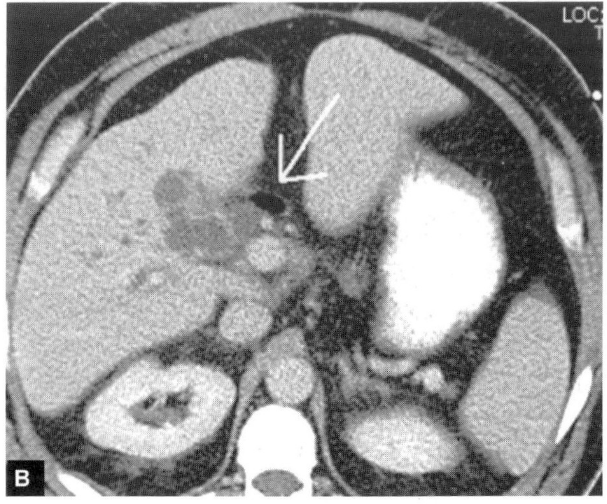

3.27B

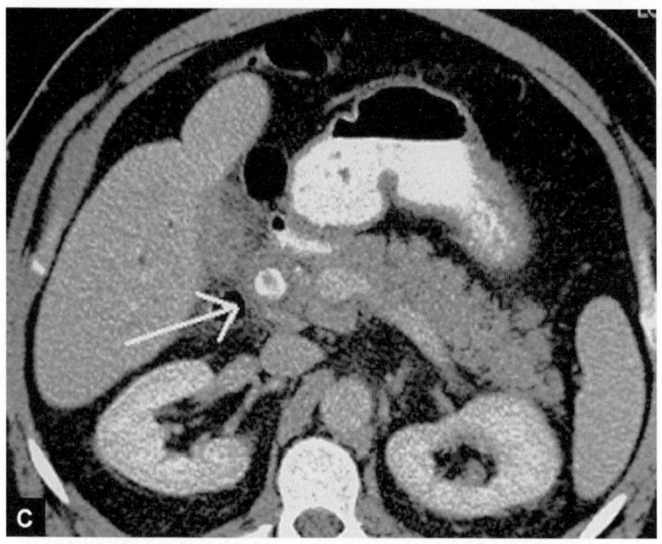

3.27C

FIGURES 3.27A to C: Patient presenting with right upper quadrant pain and suspected choledocholithiasis. (A,B) CECT, axial scans demonstrating dilated intra- and extra-hepatic bile ducts (arrows). (C) Caudal scans demonstrating a distal CBD calcified calculus with a central hypodensity (arrow)

- Calcific density stones are the easiest to detect but are not the most frequently observed type of stone (only 20% of stones display homogeneous high density). Even small stones composed of calcium bilirubinate are detectable on conventional CT. Calcified stones may be uniformly calcified (Figure 3.26) or may sometime show a central hypodensity (Figure 3.27)
- Stones composed primarily of cholesterol show lower density and thus are harder to identify

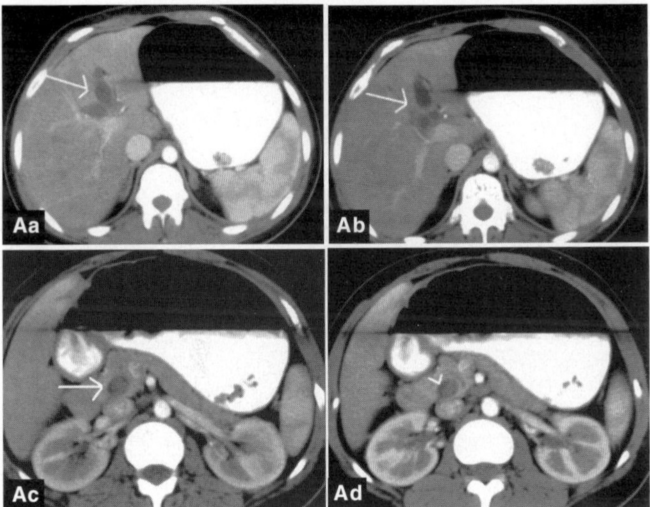

FIGURE 3.28A: Patient with history of right upper quadrant pain. (a,b) Axial scan with oral and intravenous contrast showing dilated intrahepatic bile ducts (arrows). (c,d) Caudal scans showing a mildly calcified common bile duct stone (arrow).Note the hypodense rim of bile surrounding the stone (small arrow in figure d) -representing the "target sign"

Four criteria are described by Baron on CECT:

1. *Target sign*—The calcified stone is seen as a central density surrounded by hypoattenuating bile or ampullary soft tissue (Figure 3.28A).
2. *Rim sign*—A faint rim of increased density along the margin of a low-density stone.
3. *Crescent sign*—An eccentric hyperdense calculus that is surrounded by a crescent of hypoattenuating bile or ampullary soft tissue (Figure 3.28B).
4. *Indirect signs*—Ductal dilatation with abrupt termination of the duct. However, this sign may also be seen in cholangiocarcinoma.

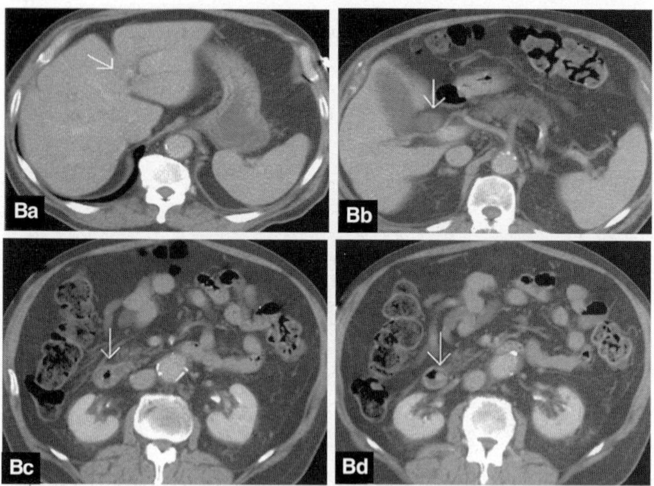

FIGURE 3.28B: Patient with history of right upper abdominal pain and suspected choledocholithiasis. (a) CECT,axial scan demonstrating dilated intra hepatic bile ducts in the left lobe (arrow). (b) Note the dilated proximal CBD at the level of the porta (arrow). (c,d) Scans at the level of the ampulla demonstrating an eccentric rounded hyperdensity sorrounded by ampullary soft tissue (arrow in figure d) likely representing a calculus –"crescentric sign".

False-positive findings:

- Enhancing vessels.
- Increased density seen within the common bile duct due to sludge or artifacts.
- Intraluminal masses

False negative findings:

- Proximal stones in minimally dilated ducts are often not suspected.
- Oral contrast material may also obscure small distal stones, especially near the ampulla of Vater (therefore,

water can be a more effective oral contrast agent in patients thought to have common bile duct stones).

- Unusual stone morphology can be misleading, such as an elongated stone resulting from bile duct cast.
- purely cholesterol stones are difficult to pick up.

CT Compared to Other Modalities[5]

ERCP: Established and effective means for diagnosing and treating choledocholithiasis. However, its invasiveness and high cost make other imaging modalities more desirable for use as the initial screening test. It also has a complication rate of 0.5 to 5%.

MRCP: The accuracy of MRCP approaches that of ERCP, but it has the disadvantage of being nontherapeutic. Artifacts may arise from surgical clips or metallic elements (these artifacts may be misinterpreted as stones). Intraductal air (which is hypointense) may mimic stones.

REFERENCES

1. Acute Biliary Disease: Initial CT and Follow-up US versus Initial US and Follow-up CT. Radiology 1999; 213: 831.
2. Tailored Helical CT Evaluation of Acute Abdomen. Radiographics 2000; 20: 725.
3. From the RSNA Refresher Courses: Imaging evaluation for acute pain in the right upper quadrant radiographics 2004; 24: 1117-35.
4. Gallbladder Stones: Imaging and intervention. Radiographics 2000; 20: 751.
5. Detection of choledocholithiasis: comparison of unenhanced helical CT and endoscopic retrograde cholangiopancreatography. Radiology 1997; 203: 753.

ACUTE PYELONEPHRITIS

Acute pyelonephritis[1] is a suppurative inflammation of the renal interstitial tissue due to an ascending urinary tract infection, usually caused by Gram-negative bacteria. It can be focal or diffuse, unilateral or bilateral. While uncomplicated acute pyelonephritis is usually diagnosed and treated on the basis of clinical findings, CT is increasingly being requested for evaluation of poor response to treatment, for detection of potential complications, and for diagnosis of underlying predisposing factors. Patients with poorly-controlled diabetes, HIV infection, and immunocompromised state are especially prone to developing complications such as a renal abscess or spread of infection to the perinephric space.

Emphysematous pyelonephritis[2]—Fulminant infection of the kidney and perirenal tissues with gas in and around the enlarged, nonfunctioning kidney with/ without formation of abscess. It is commonly seen in diabetics.

Wan et al divide emphysematous pyelonephritis into two types based on prognostic significance.

Type I emphysematous pyelonephritis is characterized by parenchymal destruction with streaky or mottled gas collections but no fluid collections. It has a 69% mortality rate.

Type II emphysematous pyelonephritis is characterized by bubbly or loculated gas within the parenchyma or collecting system with associated renal or perirenal fluid collections that are thought to represent a favorable immune response. It has an 18% mortality rate

Emphysematous pyelitis—the presence of gas limited to the renal excretory system. It is seen more commonly in women, is often associated with underlying diabetes or obstructing stone disease, and carries a mortality rate of up to 20%, which is significantly lower than that of emphysematous pyelonephritis.

It is important to differentiate it from potential noninfectious sources of gas-i.e.

i. Reflux of air from the urinary bladder due to instrumentation
ii. The presence of an ilealureterosigmoidostomy
iii. The presence of fistulae.

CT TECHNIQUE[3]

With helical/multidetector CT, there is rapid acquisition of data. This allows the kidney to be imaged in multiple phases of intravenous contrast enhancement by varying the scanning delay time.

Depending on the delay, three different phases can be imaged:

1. Cortical phase (15 sec after beginning of contrast injection), which yields the best corticomedullary differentiation.
2. parenchymal phase (45 sec after beginning of contrast injection), in which both the cortex and medullary pyramids enhance.

3. excretory phase (obtained after a delay of 5-10 min),in which pelvicalyceal contrast excretion is seen.

SCAN PROTOCOL[3]

- From the level of kidneys up to the pubic symphysis;
- 120 kVp and 140 mAs;
- Slice thickness=3 mm;
- Pitch =1:1;
- Contrast= rapid injection of iothalamate meglumine (dose of 3 mL/kg)

Note: Most important is the *parenchymal phase*—the full extent of the lesions are best depicted during the parenchymal phase. Therefore the cortical phase is generally omitted and scans are obtained in the parenchymal and excretory phases.

CT FINDINGS OF ACUTE PYELONEPHRITIS

(A) Noncontrast CT—The various findings are:

i. Normal scan—as the areas of infection are of attenuation pattern similar to the renal parenchyma and are therefore imperceptible
ii. Focal areas of low attenuation—due to edema or necrosis.
iii. Focal areas of increased attenuation—due to hemorrhage.

(B) Contrast Enhanced CT

i. Wedge-shaped, linear, or patchy areas of decreased attenuation in the renal cortex, which enhance much less compared to the normal renal parenchyma (Figure 3.29).
ii. Striation in the enhanced cortex (Figure 3.30A).
iii. Swelling or bulge in the parenchymal outline.
iv. A focal well-defined area of liquefaction with or without an enhancing rim-abscess.
v. Thickening of the renal fascia and perinephric fat stranding (Figure 3.30B).

Please note:

1. Focal acute pyelonephritis resulting in focal swelling with decreased enhancement needs to be differentiated from a tumor

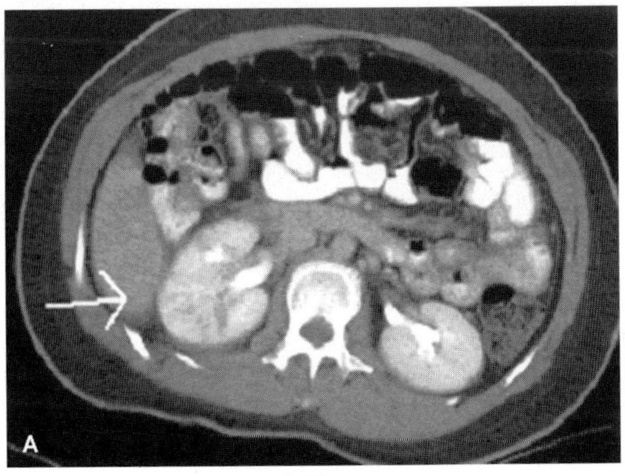

3.29A

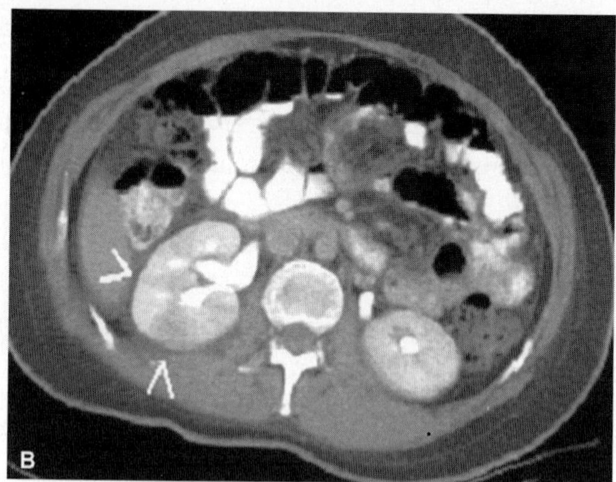

3.29B

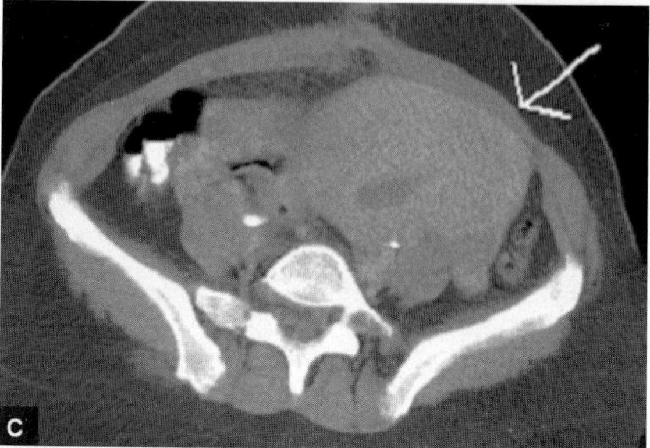

3.29C

FIGURES 3.29A to C: Postpartum female presenting with acute Right abdominal pain. (A,B) Axial scans with intravenous contrast demonstrating heterogeneous enhancement of the right kidney with ill-defined hypodensities and subtle perinephric stranding consistent with acute pyelonephtitis. (C) Caudal scan showing bulky postpartum uterus

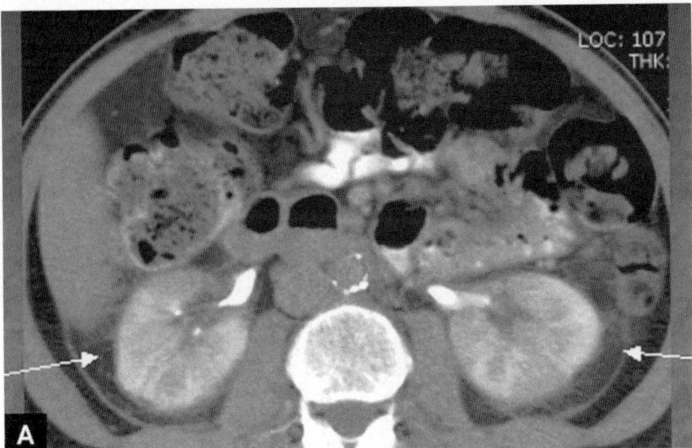

FIGURE 3.30A: Patient with history of flank pain and fever. Axial scan with intravenous contrast demonstrating heterogeneous enhancement of the kidneys with a striated appearance (arrows) and perinephric stranding bilaterally consistent with bilateral acute pyelonephritis

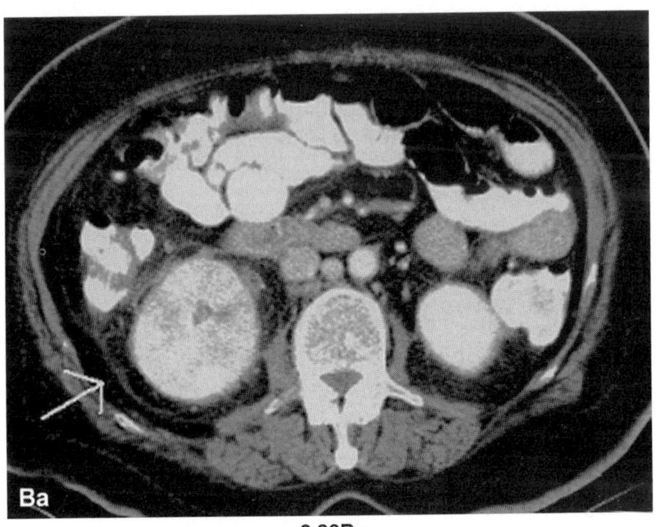

3.30Ba

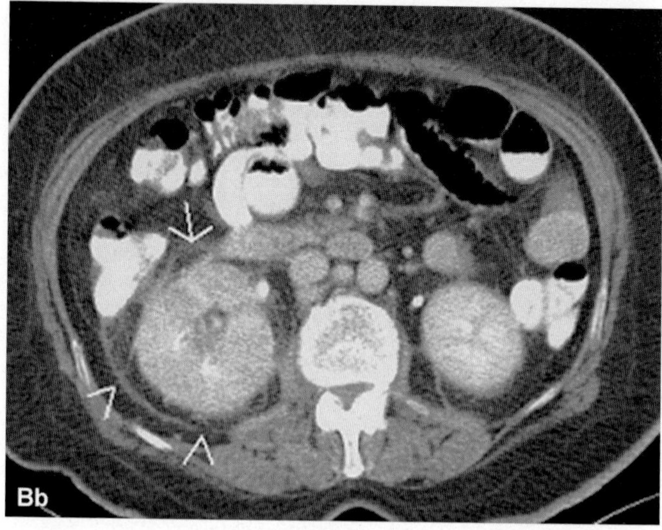

3.30Bb

FIGURE 3.30B: Patient with right flank pain and suspected pyelonephritis. (a) Axial CT scan with intravenous contrast demonstrating heterogeneously enhancing and enlarged right kidney with perinephric fat stranding. (b) Enlarged right kidney with perinephric stranding (large arrow) and thickened posterior renal fascia (small arrows) consistent with acute pyelonephritis

2. CT findings of focal swelling with decreased enhancement of confirmed acute pyelonephritis may persist for upto 6 months after treatment with antibiotics—therefore do not be misled into suspecting a neoplasm.
3. Abscess needs to be differentiated from necrotic tumor by follow-up and in equivocal cases by biopsy

ROLE OF CT

- To diagnose or exclude acute pyelonephritis.[4]

- To determine the presence of associated or causative factors—calculi and hydroureteronephrosis.
- To assess for complications like abscess formation, emphysematous pyelonephritis.
- To determine the extent and severity of involvement-focal/ diffuse, pyelonephritis /pyelitis, adjacent organ spread.

REFERENCES

1. Acute pyelonephritis: Comparison of diagnosis with ^{99m}Tc-DMSA SPECT, spiral CT, MR imaging, and power Doppler US in an experimental Pig Model[1]. Radiology 2001; 218: 101.
2. Emphysematous infections of the abdomen and pelvis: A pictorial review[1] Radiographics 2002; 22: 543.
3. Tailored Helical CT Evaluation of acute abdomen radiographics 2000; 20: 725.
4. Mimics of renal colic: Alternative diagnoses at unenhanced helical CT. Radiographics 2004; 24: S11-S28.

CHAPTER 4

CT in Bowel Obstruction

INTRODUCTION

Small and large bowel obstruction is responsible for nearly 20% of surgical admissions of patients presenting with acute abdomen.[1]

Clinical manifestations are often nonspecific and signs range from abdominal distension to signs of shock due to bowel ischemia and infarction. The early diagnosis of bowel obstruction is essential to prevent complications especially perforation and ischemia.

Plain film accuracy in evaluation of obstruction is 46-80%.[2] The possibility of closed loop obstruction and underlying ischemia has to be evaluated in order to initiate appropriate treatment. CT scan has replaced conventional imaging and can readily answer the following issues regarding bowel obstruction. It can reveal the site, level, cause of obstruction and signs of bowel ischemia, the presence of simple or closed loop obstruction. It is very important to differentiate between simple and closed loop obstruction from the point of management. Simple obstruction can be managed by conservative management, whereas in closed obstruction, surgical intervention is necessary.

CT TECHNIQUE

Scans have to be from the level of diaphragm to the symphysis pubis. Thinner sections with 5 mm interval are ideal in detecting the transition point of bowel obstruction.

In the setting of acute obstruction, where the patient is vomiting and is unable to tolerate oral contrast, scans may be obtained without oral contrast, as the intraluminal fluid and gas can serve as natural contrast agents. IV contrast is important for assessing intestinal perfusion and ischemia and evaluating the mesenteric vessels.

ETIOLOGIES OF BOWEL OBSTRUCTION

Bowel obstruction is a frequent cause of abdominal pain and accounts for 5-20% of acute surgical admissions. Adhesions are the most common cause of small bowel obstruction accounting for 60-80% (Figure 4.1). The other causes include hernias (Figure 4.2) . Approximately 95% of hernias causing bowel obstruction are external.[3] CT is excellent for detecting and characterizing bowel and mesentery in the hernia.

The other causes of small bowel obstruction include neoplasm of small bowel. Metastases are more common than primary small bowel malignancies. Miscellaneous bowel diseases like Crohn's disease, radiation enteritis, gallstone ileus, infectious enteritis and especially tuberculosis in our country constitute the remaining of the causes.

Common causes of large bowel obstruction are carcinoma (Figure 4.3), sigmoid diverticulitis and volvulus.

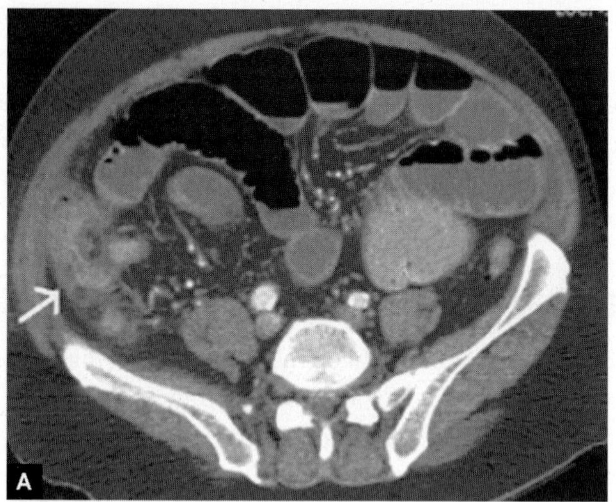

4.1A

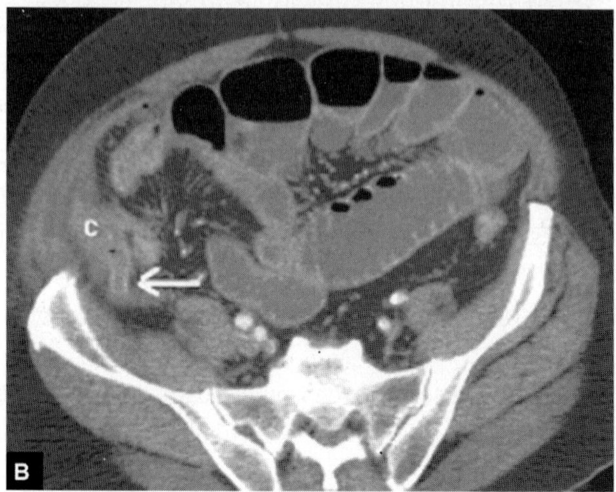

4.1B

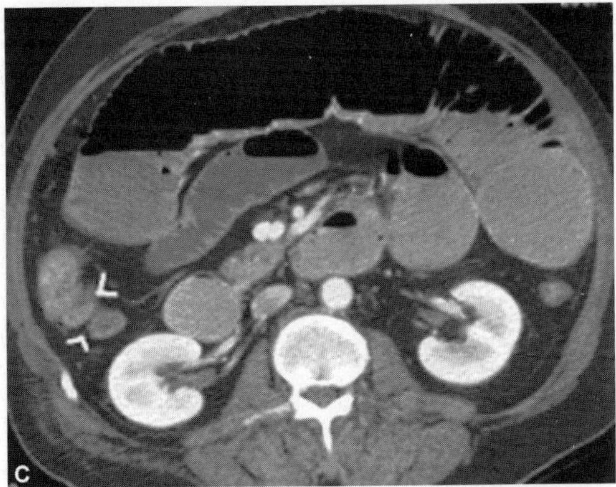

4.1C

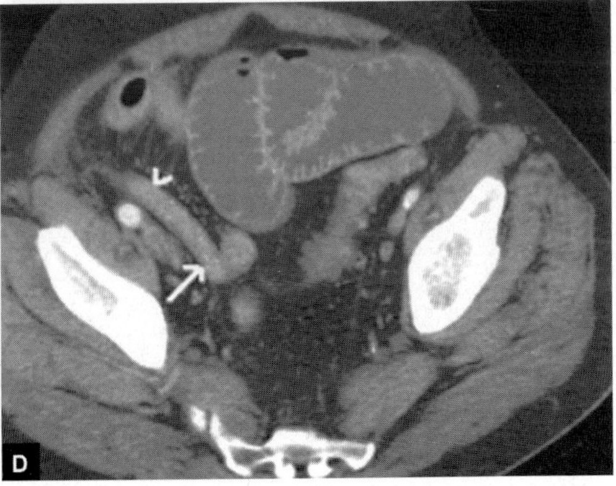

4.1D

FIGURES 4.1A to D: Small bowel obstruction secondary to inflamed appendicitis and adhesions. (A) There is cecal wall thickening with pericecal inflammation and stranding (arrow). (B) Caudal scan showing an inflamed appendix (arrow) with dilated small bowel loops. (C, D) There are multiple dilated small bowel loops with air fluid levels and collapsed distal small bowel loops (arrow heads). Consistent with high grade small bowel obstruction

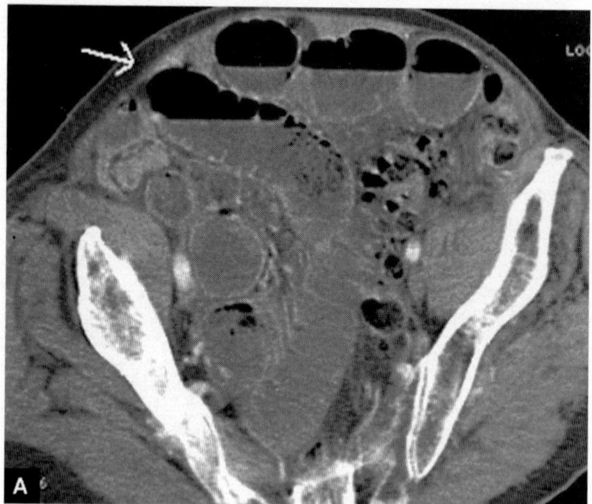

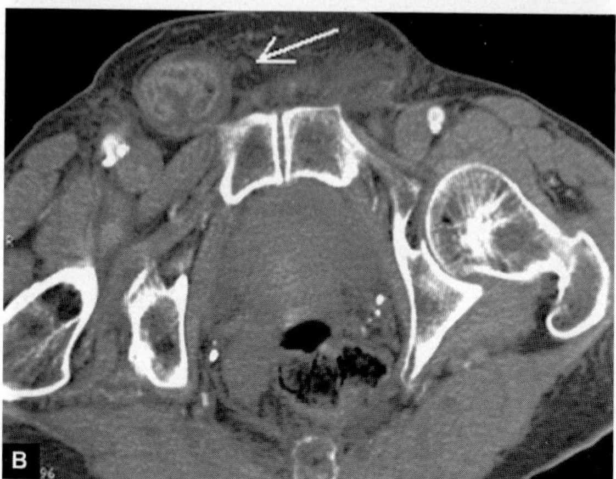

FIGURES 4.2A and B: Patient with abdominal distension and groin pain. (A) Axial scan showing multiple dilated small bowel loops with air-fluid levels. (B) Scan at the level of the inguinal region demonstrating right sided hernia containing collapsed loops within, representing the site of obstruction. This example underlies the importance of extending the scan upto the hernial sites

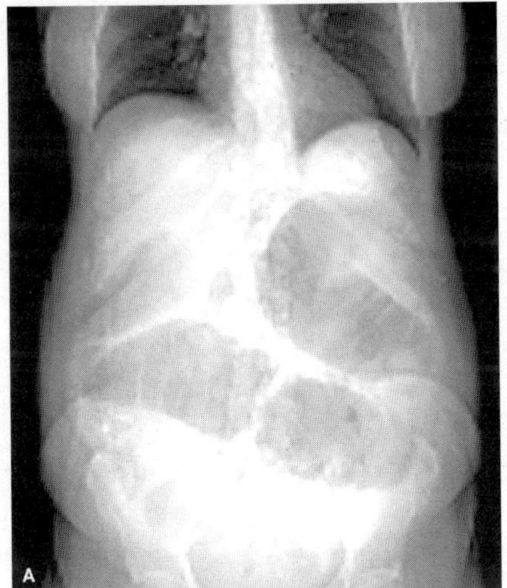

4.3A

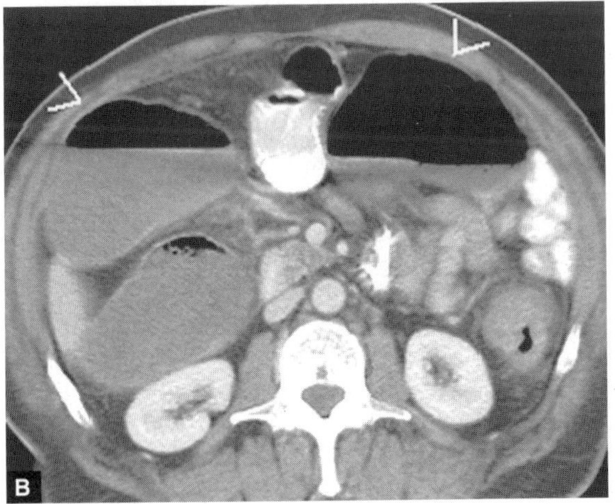

4.3B

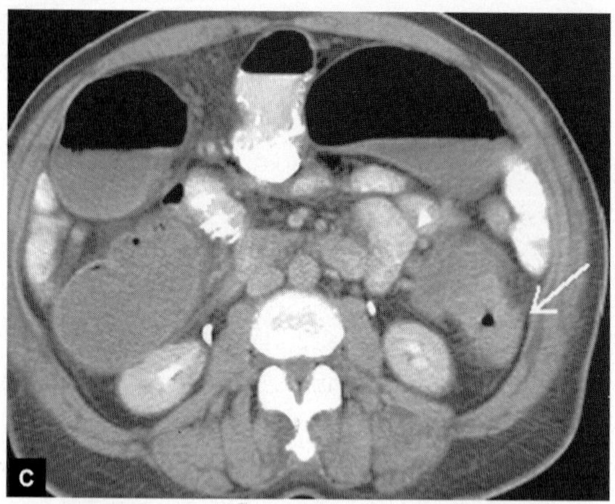

4.3C

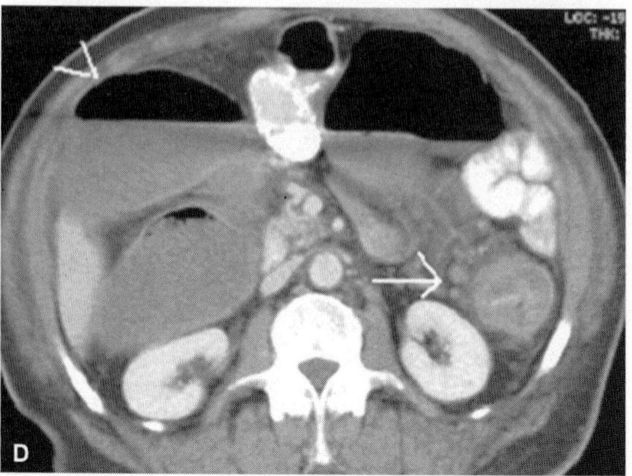

4.3D

FIGURES 4.3A to D: Patient presenting with abdominal distension and acute pain. (A) plain radiograph showing dilated colon. (B) Axial CT scan demonstrating dilated large bowel with air fluid level (small arrows). (C, D) Caudal scans demonstrating circumferential thickening of the proximal descending colon (large arrows) representing a constricting neoplasm producing large bowel obstruction

SYSTEMATIC APPROACH TO BOWEL OBSTRUCTION

The CT evaluation of bowel obstruction should be systematic.

1. The first step is confirming the presence or absence of obstruction. The usual criterion of small bowel obstruction is defined as bowel dilatation > 2.5 cm, measured from outer wall to outer wall. There should be a definite caliber change in dilated and collapsed segment with a delineation of a transition zone (careful evaluation of the transition zone can help identify the underlying cause (Figure 4.4).

   Large bowel obstruction is defined as dilatation of the large bowel greater than 6 cm or 9 cm in the cecum. Sometimes if the ileocecal valve is incompetent dilated small bowel loops may accompany a large bowel obstruction.

2. The next step is identifying the transition point and the underlying cause. It is important to differentiate between small or large bowel obstruction, as the causes, symptoms and treatment differs.

   A systematic approach begins at the rectum and then proceeds proximally towards the cecum to determine if the large or small bowel is involved. The transition point is determined by identifying a caliber change between dilated proximal and collapsed distal bowel. Although the transition point can usually be easily detected in the colon, it is often difficult in cases of small bowel obstruction.

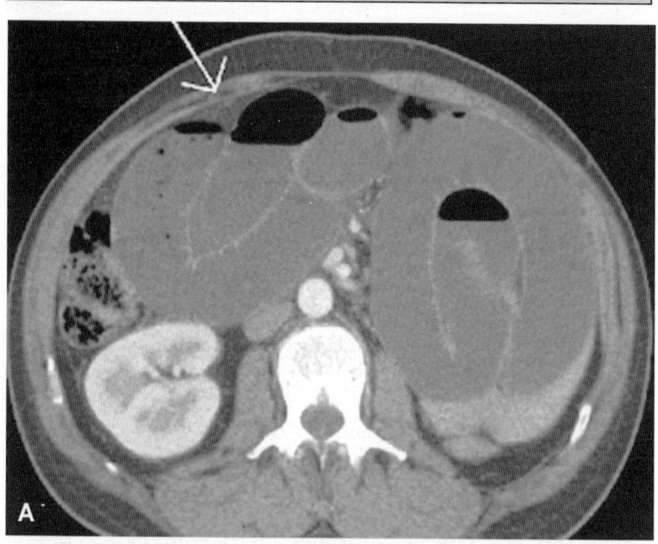

4.4A

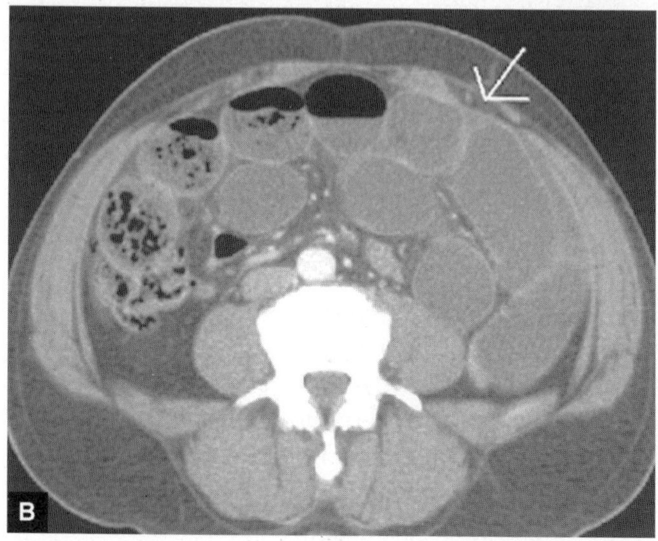

4.4B

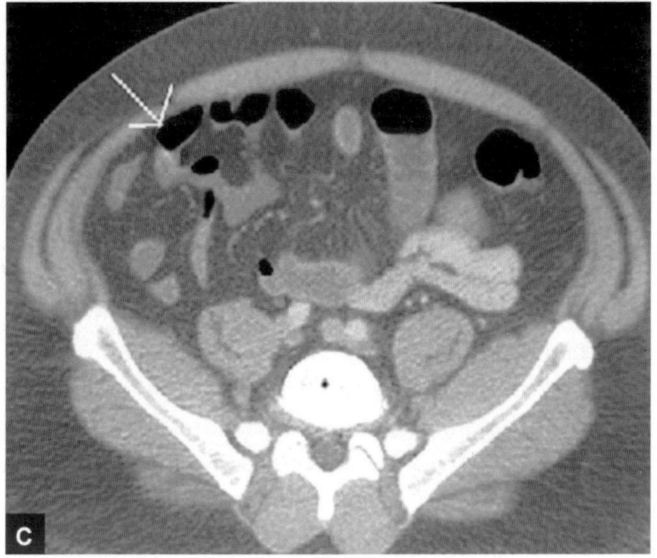

4.4C

FIGURES 4.4A to C: Patient with acute abdominal pain and distension (A,B) Axial scans with intravenous contrast showing multiple dilated loops with air fluid levels (arrows). (C) Caudal scans showing collapsed distal small bowel loops (arrow) consistent with high grade small bowel obstruction

Ideally, either the use of reformats or scrolling through the axial images in a cine mode can help in identifying the transition point. A useful CT sign that has been described in the literature can help identifying the transition zone. It is known as "Small Bowel Feces Sign".[4]

The small bowel feces sign is defined as the presence of fecal like material within the lumen of dilated loops of small bowel immediately proximal to site of obstruction (Figure 4.5). This sign tends to be most prominent at the zone of transition. It can range in length from 5-20 cm. It is commonly seen in small bowel obstruction caused by adhesions, hernias, or tumor.

The likely cause of this appearance is though to be stasis within the obstructed loop, allowing more time for fluid absorption from the bowel lumen and accumulation of undigested food particles. Careful identification of this sign may help identifying the transition point and the underlying cause.

3. After identifying the transition point, the next step is to grade the severity of the obstruction. Bowel obstruction may be partial or complete depending upon the degree of distal bowel collapse, proximal bowel dilation and the passage of contrast material beyond the transition point into the distal bowel.

   Small bowel obstruction may be graded as mild, moderate or high grade obstruction. Mild small bowel obstruction is defined as slight discrepancy between the caliber of the proximal and that of distal small bowel; moderate small bowel obstruction is discrepancy of 50% or more between the caliber of proximal and distal bowel. High grade small bowel obstruction is present if the distal small bowel and colon are collapsed. When CT findings are inconclusive, for obstruction, it is often helpful to get a delayed scan to look for the passage of contrast material.

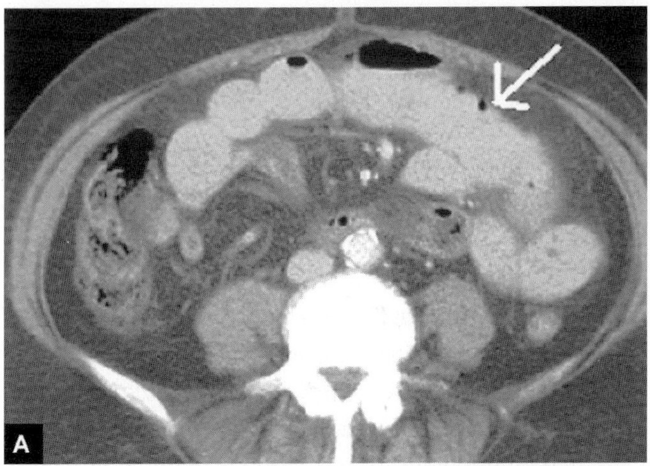

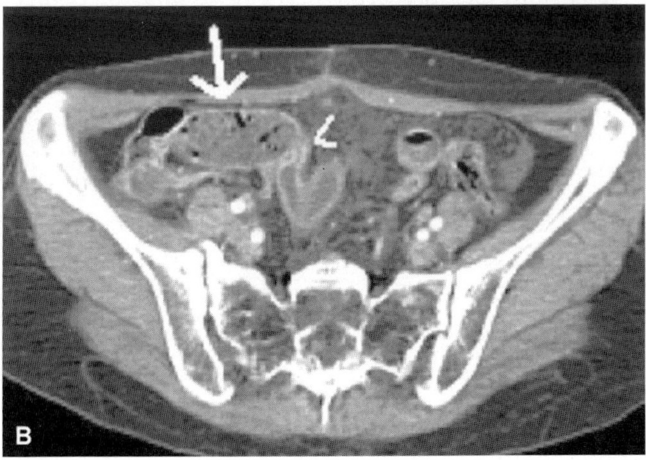

FIGURES 4.5A and B: Patient with abdominal distension and vomiting. (A) Axial scans with oral and intravenous contrast showing dilated small bowel loops(arrow). (B) Caudal scan showing the zone of transition in the distal ileum (small arrow) and the feces sign proximal to the transition(large arrow)

4. The last but the most important step is to differentiate a simple obstruction from a complicated closed loop or strangulated bowel obstruction.

   The CT features of closed loop small bowel obstruction are identified by the presence of a U-shaped or radial configuration of fluid filled dilated bowel. The adjacent mesenteric vessels may be seen to be converging towards the point of obstruction (Figure 4.6). Also at the site of obstruction, there may be a whirl sign,[5] a beak sign or triangular configuration of adjacent collapsed loops. The presence of a whirl indicates a twist in mesentery

   The triangular segments represent the afferent and efferent entry points or the torsion site.

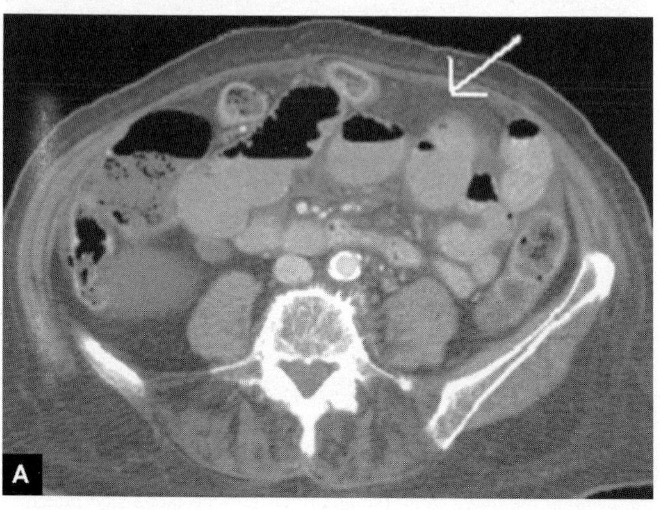

4.6A

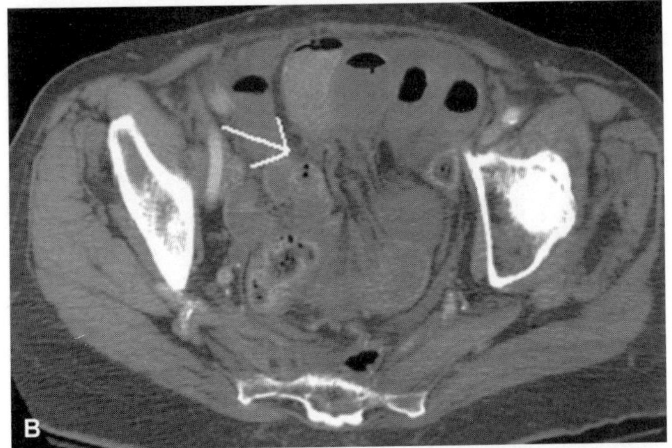

4.6B

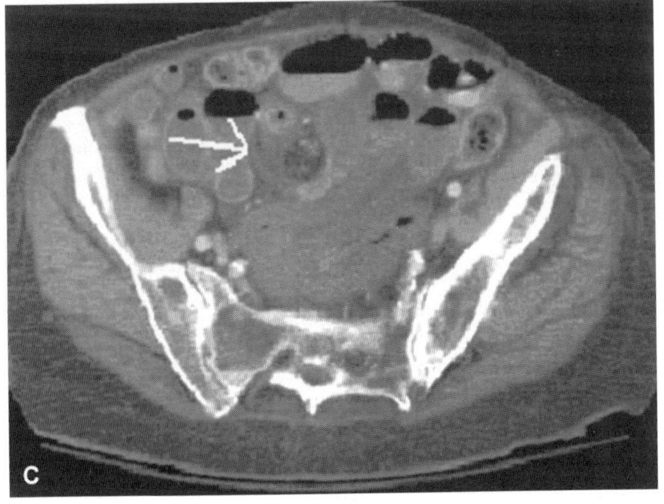

4.6C

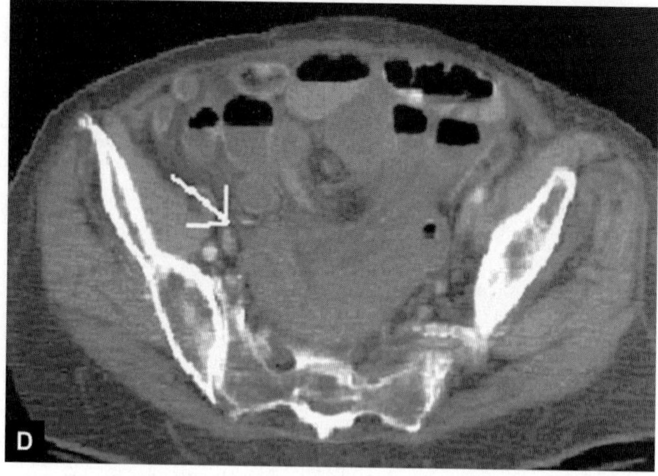

4.6D

FIGURES 4.6A to D: Patient with suspected small bowel obstruction (A) Axial scan with oral and intravenous contrast showing multiple dilated small bowel loops (arrow). (B) There is abnormal arrangement of small bowel loops in the pelvis. (C) Caudal scan showing a twist in the mesentery(arrow). (D) A segment of a loop in the pelvis is thickened(arrow) with surrounding stranding suggestive of ischemic changes within the thickened segment

Bowel strangulation manifests as mesenteric stranding adjacent to the affected loop usually due to congestive changes or hemorrhage within mesenteric fat.

Finally, when ischemic changes occur, there may be bowel wall thickening, a target sign or there may be poor or delayed enhancement of the involved bowel. Obstruction to venous outflow is usually the cause of ischemia in bowel obstruction. It usually results from increase in intraluminal pressure from progressive bowel dilation.

Intestinal ischemia and infarction are the major causes of morbidity and mortality in patients with bowel obstruction. Hence, careful evaluation is essential to differentiate between a simple or complicated bowel obstruction

In conclusion, CT is an effective tool in evaluation of bowel obstruction. It can confirm the presence of obstruction, site of obstruction, the underlying cause, the severity and finally differentiate between simple or complicated bowel obstruction. The various signs and appearances described in this chapter help in correct diagnosis and initiate appropriate treatment.

POINTS TO REMEMBER

1. Always measure the lumen diameter, never eyeball, early obstruction may be missed.
2. Try to identify the small bowel feces sign in case of small bowel obstruction to locate the transition.
3. Always look for hernial sites to avoid missing the probable cause of obstruction.
4. Look for signs of complicated bowel obstruction like whirl sign, signs of ischemia.
5. Differentiate between a simple or closed loop obstruction, as management varies.

REFERENCES

1. Welch JP. General consideration and mortality in bowel obstruction. In: Welch JP, Ed. Bowel Obstruction: Differential Diagnosis and Clinical Manifestation. Philadelphia: Saunders, 1990: 59-95.
2. Maglinte DD, Reyes Bl, Harmon BH, et al. Reliability and role of plain film radiography and CT in the diagnosis of small bowel obstruction. AJR 1996; 167: 1451-5.
3. Herlinger H, Rubesin SE. Obstruction. In : Gore RM, Levine MS, Laufer 1 (Eds): Textbook of Gastrointestinal Radiology, Vol 1. Philadelphia: Saunders, 1994; 931-66.
4. Mayo-Smith WW, Wittenberg J, Bennet GL, Gervais DA, Gazelle GS, Mueller PR. The CT small bowel feces sign: description and clinical significance. Clin Radial 1995; 50: 765-7.
5. Fisher JK. Computed tomographic diagnosis of volvulus in intestinal malrotation. Radiology 1981; 140: 145-6.

GALLSTONE ILEUS

INTRODUCTION

Gallstone ileus is an important, though infrequent cause of mechanical bowel obstruction, affecting elderly patients who often have other significant medical conditions.

The diagnosis is often delayed since symptoms may be intermittent and investigations fail to identify the cause of the obstruction.

Gallstone ileus continues to be associated with relatively high rates of morbidity and mortality.

INCIDENCE

Less than 0.5 percent of patients with cholelithiasis present with the complication of gallstone ileus. The term gallstone ileus is actually a misnomer, the more accurate descriptor would be gallstone induced small bowel obstruction. Gallstone ileus accounts for 20 to 25 percent of non-strangulated small bowel obstruction,[1] in patients over age 65. Thus, gallstone ileus should always be in the differential diagnosis when evaluating an elderly person with intestinal obstruction.

The average age of patients with gallstone ileus is 70 years, Females are affected 3 to 16 times more commonly than males

ETIOPATHOGENESIS

The usual means of gallstone entry into the bowel is through a biliary-enteric fistula, which complicates 2 to 3 percent of all cases of cholelithiasis with associated episodes of cholecystitis.

Sixty percent are cholecystoduodenal fistulas, but cholecystocolonic and cholecystogastric fistulas can also result in gallstone ileus.[1,3]

The following sequence is responsible for most cases of fistula formation. Pericholecystic inflammation after cholecystitis leads to the development of adhesions between the biliary and enteric systems. Pressure necrosis by the gallstone against the biliary wall then causes erosion and fistula formation. In addition, gallstone ileus has occurred after endoscopic sphincterotomy.

In the majority of cases the gallstone will pass through the intestinal tract without difficulty; however, with a stone larger than 2.5 cm, intestinal obstruction is likely. The point of obstruction (2) is generally in the ileum or at the ileocecal valve (76%), in the duodenum (21%) or sigmoid colon (2%). The site of communication between the biliary tract and the intestine is most commonly at the duodenum or colon. Gallstone obstruction in the colon will usually be at the site of a previous disease process such as sigmoid diverticulosis, or at a surgical anastomosis.[4] Gastric outlet obstruction may result if the stone remains in the duodenum (Bouveret's Syndrome).

CLINICAL FEATURES

Typically, gallstone ileus presents as unexplained gradual onset of small bowel obstruction. Rarely, the stone may traverse the small bowel and obstruct the large bowel. In both, pain, distension, constipation and vomiting are present to varying degrees. Additionally, a mass may be felt in the right upper quadrant.

DIAGNOSIS

Classically, abdominal radiography reveals a triad of features,

- Gas in the biliary tree:
  40% of cases
- A gallstone in the intestine:
  often at the ileocecal junction
- Small bowel obstruction
- The radiographic triad of small bowel obstruction, pneumobilia and ectopic gallstone on abdominal plain radiograph is also described with CT imaging (Figures

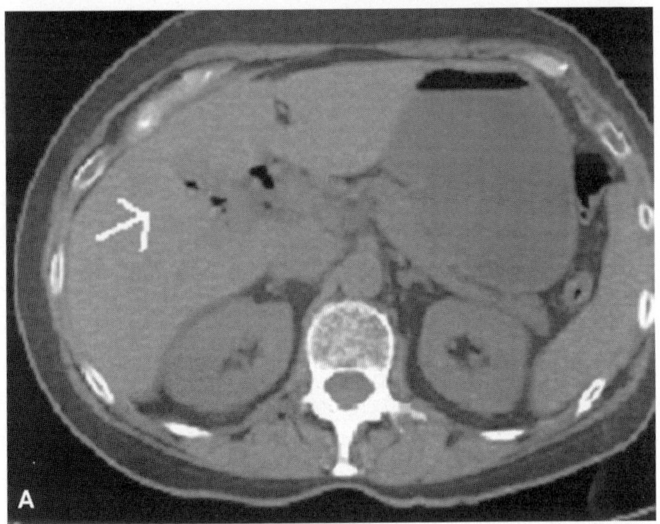

4.7A

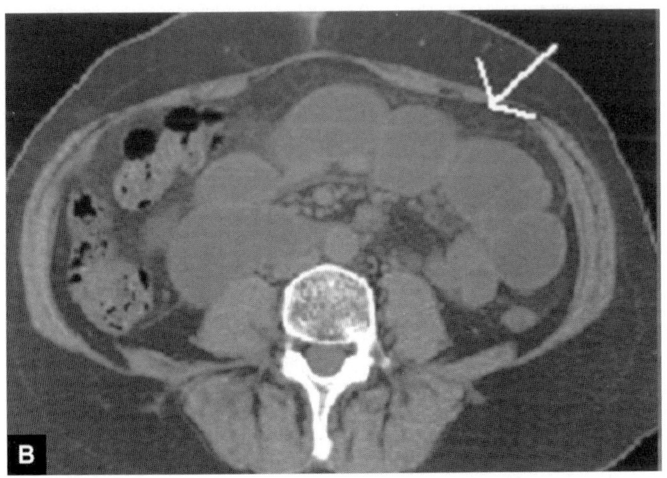

4.7B

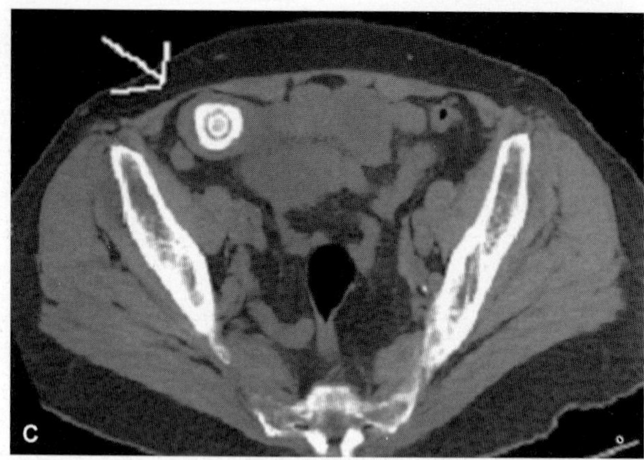

4.7C

FIGURES 4.7A to C: Patient presenting with abdominal distension and vomiting. (A) Axial non contrast scan showing air within the gallbladder. (B) There are multiple dilated small bowel loops. (C) Caudal scans showing a large calculus in the distal ileum consistent with gallstone ileus

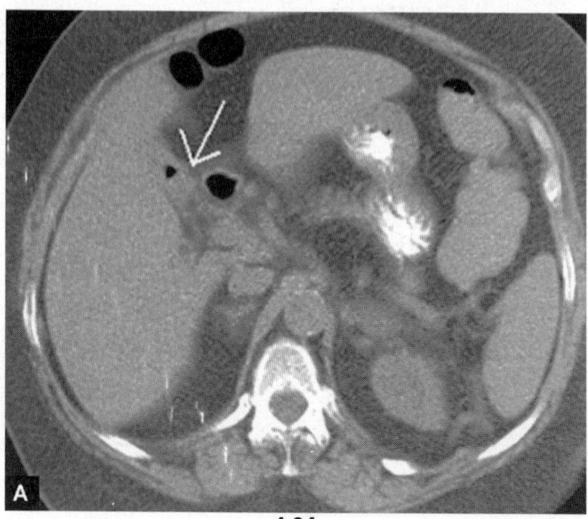

4.8A

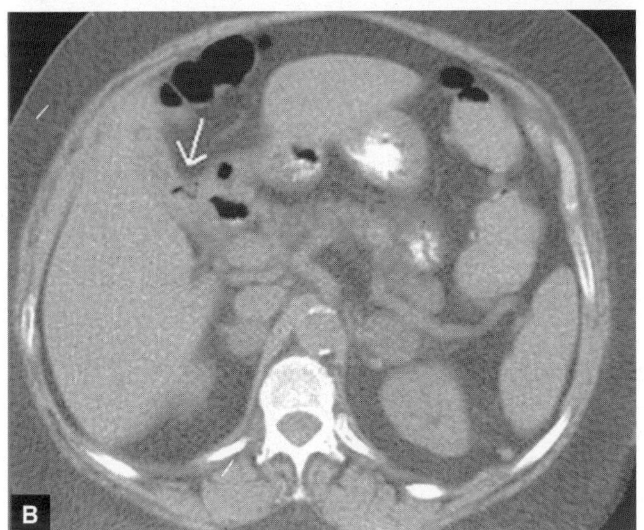

4.8B

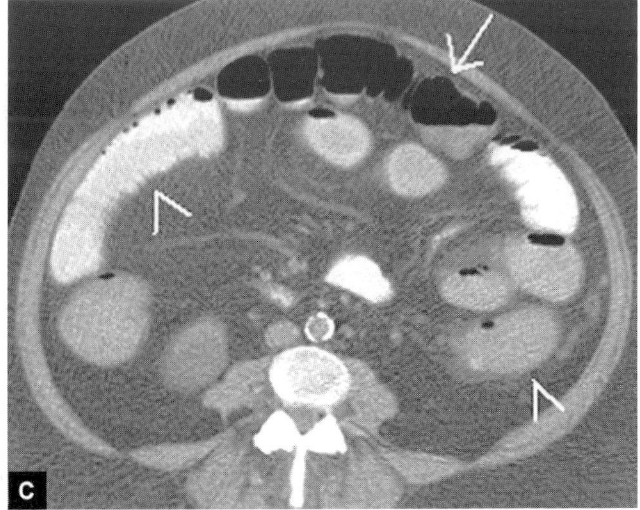

4.8C

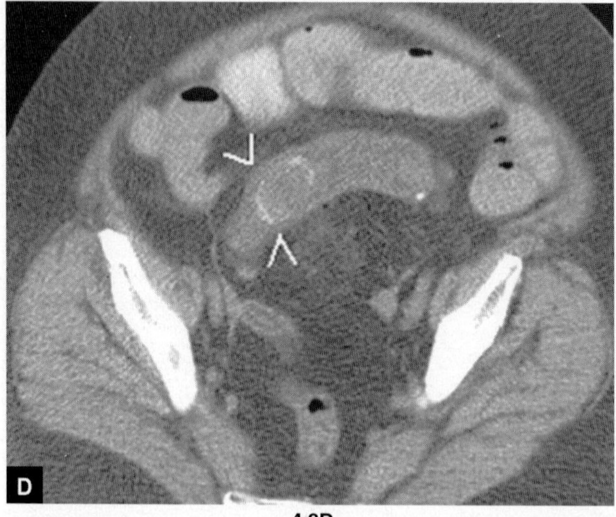

4.8D

FIGURES 4.8A to D: Patient presenting with abdominal distension and signs of obstruction. (A) Axial scans with oral contrast showing air within the gallbladder (arrow). (B) Sequential image showing fistulous communication between gallbladder and duodenum (arrow). (C) There are multiple dilated large and small bowel loops (arrow). (D) A rounded hyperdensity is seen in the sigmoid colon consistent with a calculus within the sigmoid colon and producing small and large bowel obstruction

4.7 and 4.8). Because of the better resolution of CT compared with abdominal radiography, its increased sensitivity as compared with plain film radiography in the detection of all three signs of gallstone ileus and its recent increased availability in the emergency setting, it has become the modality of choice in the imaging of this condition.

Additionally, a barium meal may show reflux into the gallbladder and biliary tree through a fistula, but is best avoided when surgery is contemplated.

REFERENCES

1. Reisner RM, Cohen JR. Gallstone ileus: review of 1001 reported cases. Am Surg 1994; 60: 441-6.
2. Maglinte DDT, Balthazar EJ, Kelvin FM, Megibow AJ. The role of radiology in the diagnosis of small-bowel obstruction. Am J Roentgenol 1997; 168: 1171-80.
3. Swift SE, Spencer JA. Gallstone Ileus : CT findings, Clin Radiol 1998; 53: 451-4.
4. Scarpa Francis J, Borges James, Mullen David. Gallstone Ileus. Am J Surg 2000; 180: 99.

CHAPTER 5

CT in the Evaluation of Intestinal Volvulus

INTRODUCTION

Bowel obstruction is a common cause of emergency surgical presentation. The more common causes are well known and may be treated conservatively. However not all cause of bowel obstruction are as simple, as some of the less common causes require immediate diagnosis and treatment, failing which they may progress to ischemia and gangrene. Among such causes is bowel volvulus. Volvulus is a condition wherein there is a twist of the intestine on its mesenteric axis, resulting in complete or partial obstruction. Volvulus can involve the small or large bowel. In this section we will describe the CT findings with illustrations.

SMALL BOWEL VOLVULUS

Small bowel volvulus is a rare but life-threatening surgical emergency. There are two types depending on the etiology.

1. *Primary:* Usually occurs in children and young adults. The usual cause is unclear. However, large quantities of fiber diet after prolonged fasting or increased gut motility may have a role.
2. *Secondary:* Secondary small bowel volvulus usually occurs later with a peak incidence in the 6th-8th decades.[1] The predisposing factors are bands, adhesions, internal hernias and prior surgery. The suggested mechanism involves obstruction of a small bowel loop

at two fixed points by one of these predisposing conditions. As the loop fills with fluid , peristalsis causes it to twist around its mesentery. Small bowel volvulus presents with features of intestinal obstruction. The most common finding is central abdominal pain, out of proportion to the degree of obstruction. Associated symptoms include nausea, vomiting and abdominal distension. As small bowel volvulus involves a twist in the mesentery, there is compression of the mesenteric vascular supply to the bowel resulting in ischemia and bowel infarction. Thus, early preoperative investigation and surgery are required if bowel infarction is to be prevented.

The plain film radiologic features of small bowel volvulus are nondiagnostic and show nonspecific features of small bowel obstruction with either air distended loops or a gasless abdomen with fluid-filled bowel loops. CT has been proved to be effective in diagnosing complex small bowel obstruction and bowel ischemia with high level of sensitivity and accuracy described in the literature.[2].

CT FEATURES OF SMALL BOWEL VOLVULUS

The CT features of small bowel volvulus are identification of a complex closed loop obstruction, wherein there is a radial or U-shaped configuration of the distended loops. The other key findings are the presence of a twist in the mesentery manifesting as a Whirl.

The 'Whirl sign' is highly suggestive of small bowel volvulus. The Whirl sign was first described by Fisher.[3] This sign occurs when afferent and efferent loops rotate around a fixed point of obstruction, which results in twisted mesentery along the axis of rotation (Figure 5.1).

These twisted loops of bowel and branching mesenteric vessels create swirling strands of soft tissue attenuation within a background of mesenteric fat, giving the appearance of a hurricane on a weather map. Thus the presence of the Whirl sign is highly suggestive of small bowel volvulus and should raise suspicion for a complicated bowel obstruction. In addition, other complications resulting from closed loop obstruction have to be carefully looked for.

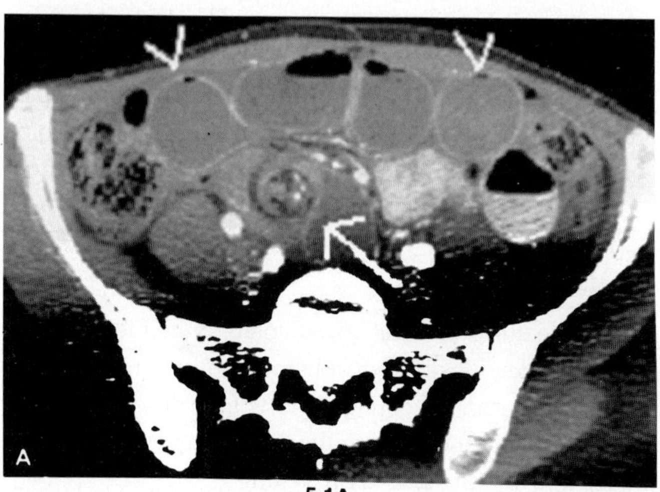

5.1A

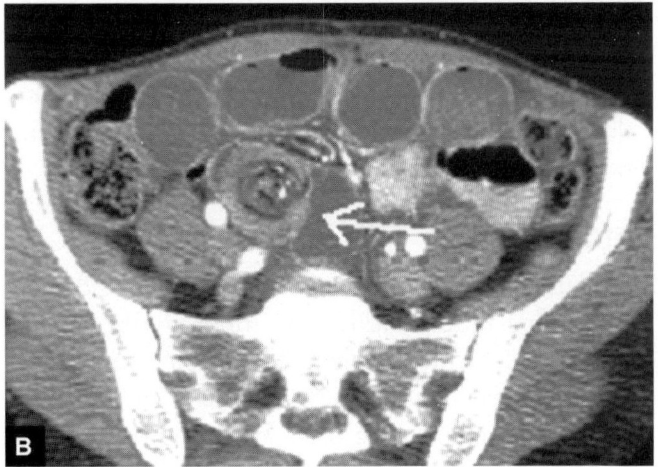

5.1B

FIGURES 5.1A and B: The CT "whirl sign". (A,B) Axial scans in a case of small bowel volvulus showing the CT whirl sign(large arrows) and dilated small bowel loops (small arrows). The CT "Whirl sign" occurs when afferent and efferent loops rotate around a fixed point of obstruction, which result in twisted mesentery along the axis of rotation. These twisted loops of bowel and branching mesenteric vessels create swirling strands of soft tissue attenuation within a background of mesenteric fat, giving the appearance of a hurricane on a weather map

LARGE BOWEL VOLVULUS

Volvulus of the colon represents the third most common cause of colonic obstruction after carcinoma and diverticulitis.

Colonic volvulus generally occurs when a non-retroperitoneal segment of the colon twists on its mesenteric axis. This results in obstruction and eventually ischemia from compromise of the vascular supply as well as luminal distension with increased wall tension and decreased transmural blood flow .Volvulus occurs in those portions of colon possessing a mesentery, including the sigmoid colon, cecum, transverse colon and rarely the splenic flexure.[4]

ETIOLOGY

The causative or contributing factors to the development of volvulus may include high fiber diets, chronic constipation, and altered colonic motility as a result of aging or medication (elderly and psychiatric patients) . The most common cause of large bowel obstruction in pregnancy is cecal volvulus, probably as a result of the gravid uterus elevating the cecum.

CLINICAL FEATURES

Patients with colonic volvulus typically present with abdominal distension and constipation. Nausea and vomiting occurs with increased duration. In severe cases patients may present with shock suggesting perforation or bowel gangrene.

The diagnosis of colonic volvulus can be generally be suspected on conventional abdominal radiographs and can be confirmed with barium enema. Various signs and appearances have been well-described. However, they offer no information about complications such as bowel ischemia or other abnormalities outside the bowel wall. Also the findings on plain radiographs could be obscured if there is closed loop obstruction with fluid filled loops, or obscured by air-distended bowel. CT is usually the imaging technique of choice for patients presenting with acute abdomen.[5]

CT can reveal the presence and location of volvulus, and allow early identification of potentially fatal complications, such as ischemia and perforation.

CT OF CECAL VOLVULUS

Cecal volvulus accounts for 11% of all intestinal volvulus, usually occurring in the adults (30-60 yrs).

In cecal volvulus, the cecum twists in the axial plane, rotating clockwise or anticlockwise around its long axis to lie in the right lower quadrant, or twist and invert, occupying the left upper quadrant. It may also fold upward anteriorly without any torsion known as 'cecal bascule'. Cecal bascule is commonly seen as a dilated loop in the mid abdomen.

CT SIGNS OF CECAL VOLVULUS

On CT, cecal volvulus is suggested by the extreme dilatation of the cecum (Figure 5.2) A specific CT sign for volvulus is the "whirl", which has been described in volvulus of the midgut, cecum and sigmoid colon.[6,7]

The whirl is composed of tightly twisted bowel, mesentery and vessels. The tightness of the whirl is proportionate to the degree of rotation. CT can also shows signs of strangulation like circumferential thickening of

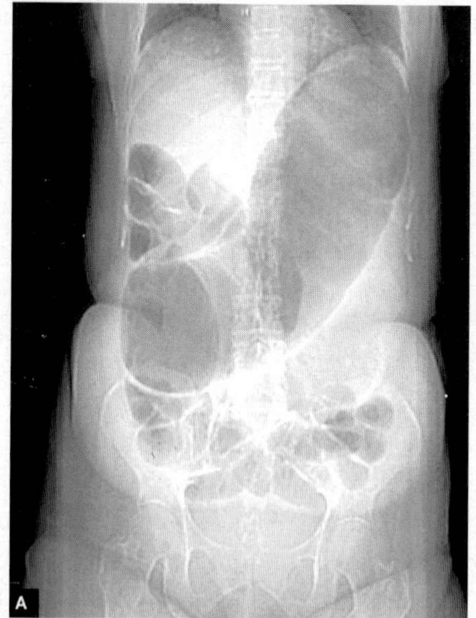

5.2A

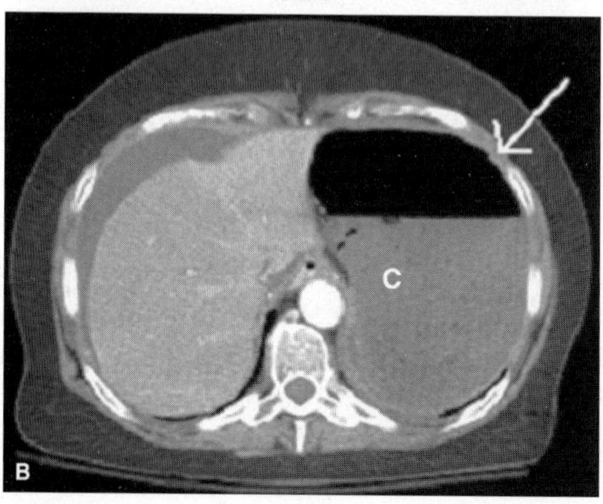

5.2B

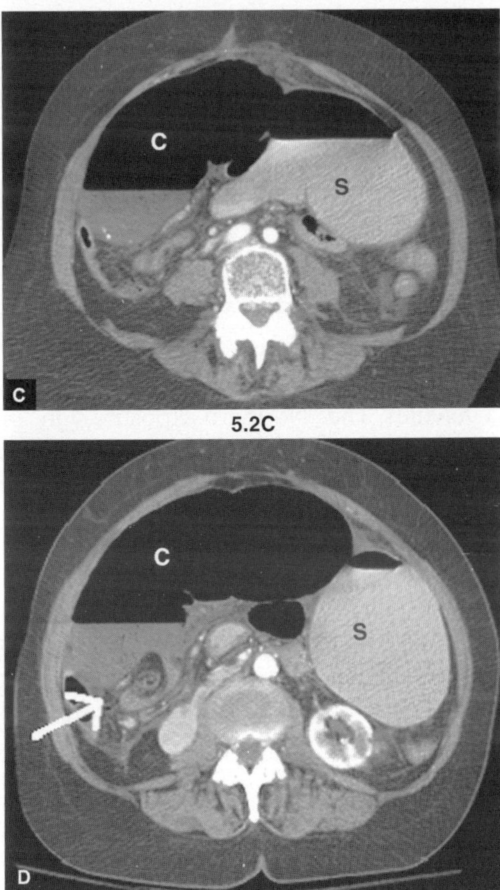

FIGURES 5.2A to D: Patient presenting with abdominal distension and vomiting and suspected bowel obstruction. (A) Topogram demonstrating a gas-filled dilated structure in the mid abdomen. (B,C) The cecum in markedly dilated and lies in the upper and left abdomen close to the stomach. (D) Caudal scan showing dilated cecum and twist at the base of cecum with positive whirl sign (large arrow) consistent with cecal volvulus C=cecum,S=stomach

bowel wall, intestinal pneumatosis, mesenteric stranding and hemorrhagic fluid.[8]

SIGMOID VOLVULUS

In sigmoid volvulus, the sigmoid colon twists along the mesentery of the inferior mesenteric artery. The mean age is in the 7th decade. Generally, ischemic changes are less frequent in cases of sigmoid volvulus as compared to cecal volvulus.

Plain abdominal radiographs are usually diagnostic in sigmoid volvulus. The "Northern exposure sign" in which the sigmoid colon is cephalad to the transverse colon has also been described.[9] As previously mentioned CT in addition can provide information about complication of bowel ischemia and perforation.

The specific CT sign for volvulus is the 'whirl sign' as described earlier (Figure 5.3). CT can also demonstrate signs of strangulation. CT is more specific than barium in delineating the presence, cause, level and degree of bowel obstruction and associated abnormalities outside the bowel.

In summary, volvulus of the colon, may occur when there is a twist in the mesocolon. Early diagnosis is essential to prevent potential complications of volvulus like bowel ischemia, gangrene and perforation. CT can accurately identify the site and degree of obstruction. The presence of whirl sign and associated bowel dilatation determine the diagnosis of volvulus. CT can also show signs of strangulation and perforation and help in planning treatment.

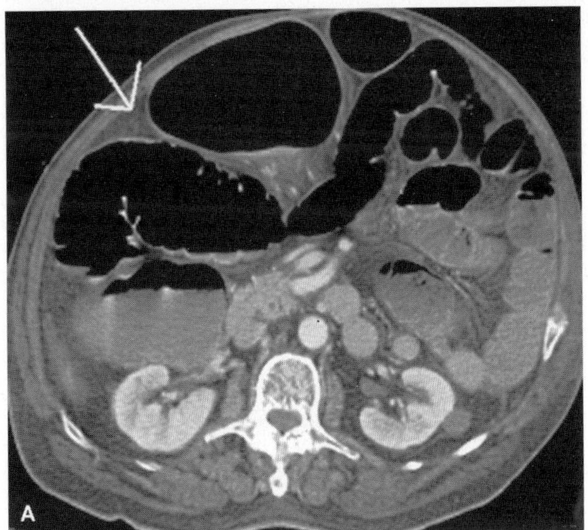

5.3A

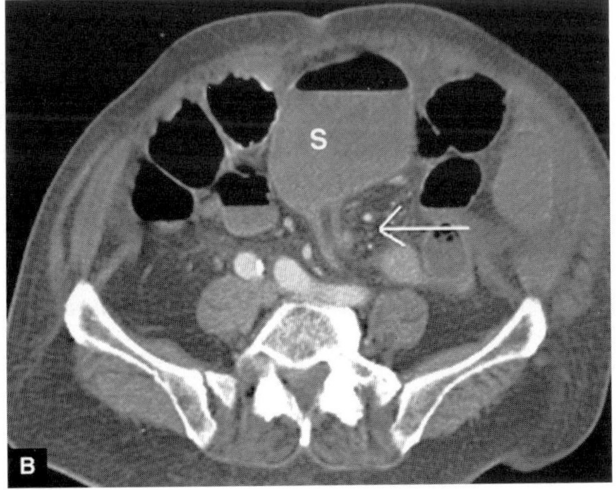

5.3B

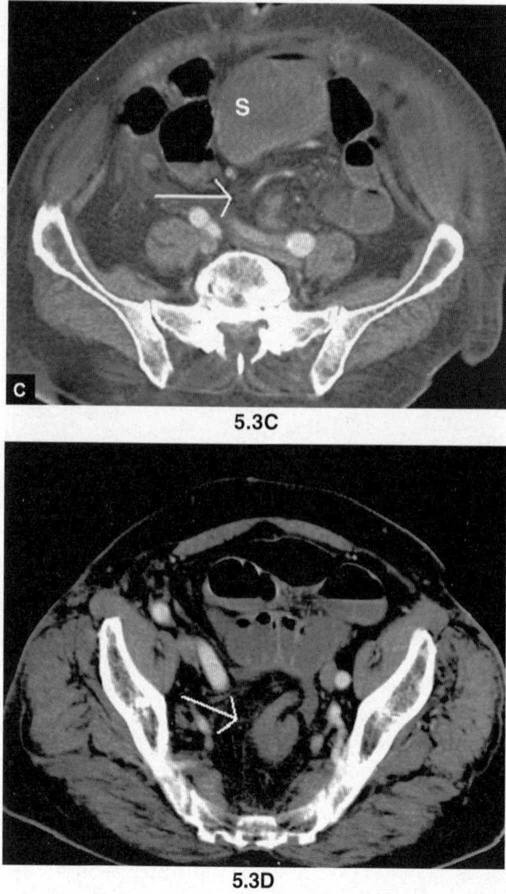

5.3C

5.3D

FIGURES 5.3A to D: An elderly patient presented with abdominal distension and constipation. (A) Axial scans showing dilated large and small bowel loops (arrow). (B) Note the dilated sigmoid colon in the mid abdomen and the Nondilated afferent and efferent limbs of the twisted sigmoid colon(arrow). (C) Caudal scan showing the twisted sigmoid mesocolon with the whirl (large arrow) consistent with sigmoid volvulus. (D) The rectum is collapsed(arrow). S=sigmoid colon

POINTS TO REMEMBER

1. Volvulus is a twist in mesentery - look for signs of twist, "whirl sign" is highly suggestive of small or large bowel volvulus.
2. Look for complications of volvulus like closed loop obstruction in small bowel volvulus, strangulation and ischemia in colonic volvulus.

REFERENCES

1. Welch GH, Ander, JR. Volvulus of the small intestine in adults. World J Surg 1986; 10: 496-9.
2. Balthazar EJ, Liebskind ME, Macari M. Intestinal ischemia in patients in whom small bowel obstruction is suspected; evaluation of accuracy, limitation, and clinical implication of CT in diagnosis. Radiology 1997; 205: 519-22.
3. Fisher JK. Computed tomographic diagnosis of volvulus in intestinal malrotation. Radiology 1981; 140: 145-6.
4. Mindelzum RE, Stone JM. Volvulus of the splenic flexure; radiographic features. Radiology 1991; 181: 221-3.
5. Perrer RS, Kumberger LE. Cecal volvulus. AJR 1998; 171:860.
6. Frank AJ, Goffner LB, Fruaff AA, Losada RA. Cecal volvulus: The CT whirl sign, Abdominal imaging 1993; 18: 288-289.
7. Catalano O. Computed tomographic appearance of sigmoid volvulus. Abdom Imaging 1996; 21: 314-7.
8. Balthazar EJ, Birnbaum BA, Megibow AJ, et al. Closed loop and strangulating intestinal obstruction: CT signs. Radiology 1992: 185: 769-75.
9. Javors BR, Baker Sr, Miller JA. The Northern exposure sign: a newly described finding in sigmoid volvulus. AJR 1999; 173: 571-4.

CHAPTER 6

Abdominal Wall Hernias and Role of CT

INTRODUCTION

Abdominal wall hernias account for most of external hernias. Patients may present with acute abdominal pain, relating to complications of hernia like incarceration, strangulation or bowel obstruction. Although diagnosis is usually made at physical examination, clinical diagnosis may be difficult in patients with severe pain or obesity. Hence, imaging may be of value to correct diagnosis.

Conventional radiographs and barium were earlier used in confirming abdominal wall hernias, however the complications of hernia like incarceration, bowel obstruction, or strangulation.cannot be accurately evaluated on radiographs. CT has evolved as the ideal technique to evaluate hernias. CT can accurately identify abdominal wall hernias, characterize bowel and mesentery in the hernia sac. CT can differentiate hernia from other abdominal masses (tumors, abscess, hematomas) , detect complication like incarceration, bowel obstruction and strangulation. Approximately 28% of obstruction caused by hernias is complicated by strangulation and ischemia.[1]

CT is also useful in evaluating postsurgical patients and markedly obese patient in determining the shape, location and content of abdominal wall hernias. Further more CT with Multiplanar reformats and 3D images can precisely delineate hernia type, location, size and shape.

Hernias can be classified as –

A. Groin hernias
   i. Inguinal.
   ii. Femoral.

B. Ventral hernias
   i. Midline defect
   ii. Lateral defect
   iii. Posterior defect
C. Incisional hernias
D. Miscellaneous hernias
   i. Richter's hernia
   ii. Obturator hernia

GROIN HERNIAS

INGUINAL HERNIAS

Inguinal hernias are the most common abdominal wall hernias constituting about 60%.[2] They result from herniation through a patent processus vaginalis and are located lateral to the inferior epigastric vessels. In adults they are caused by acquired weakness and dilation of internal inguinal ring.[3] CT can depict the size, show the contents and complications like incarceration and strangulation (Figure 6.1). The CT signs of strangulation are

1. Mesenteric stranding.
2. Wall thickening.
3. Poor bowel wall enhancement, free air, or fluid in the hernial sac.

FEMORAL HERNIAS

They are less frequent and occur commonly in women. They arise from a defect in the attachment of transversalis

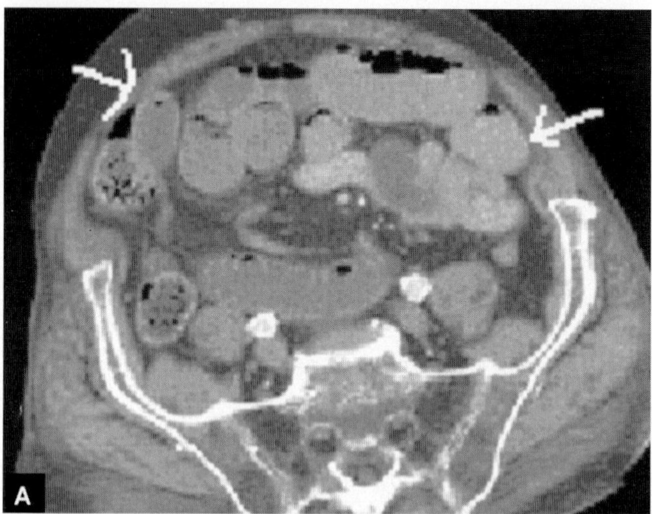

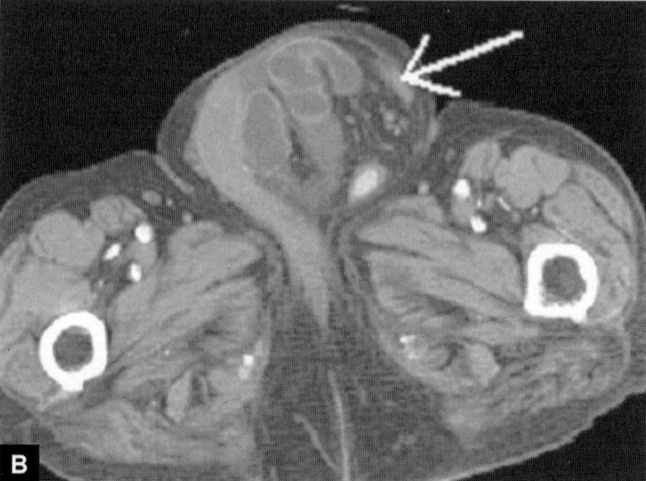

FIGURES 6.1A and B: A case of left inguinal hernia producing small bowel obstruction. (A) Axial scan showing multiple dilated small bowel loops. (B) Scan at the level of the left groin showing a inguinal hernia with obstructed loops

fascia to the pubic tubercle and occur medial to the femoral vein. They are difficult to differentiate from inguinal hernias and have a high tendency to incarcerate.[4]

VENTRAL HERNIAS

Ventral hernias include all hernias through anterior or lateral abdominal wall defect.

Midline hernias include umbilical and epigastric hernias. Although umbilical hernias are commonly seen in neonates, they spontaneously close in childhood. In adults, they are acquired and occur more commonly in women. The risk factors are multiple pregnancies, obesity, intra-abdominal masses.[3,4]

Umbilical hernia has a high incidence of incarceration and strangulation. A paraumbilical hernia is a defect in the linear alba in the region of umbilicus and related to diastasis of the rectus abdominis muscle.

Epigastric hernias are uncommon. They appear on the linea alba between the umbilicus and the xyphoid process. They usually occur in obese patient and their symptoms may mimic gallbladder disease or peptic ulcer disease.

LATERAL DEFECTS

Spigelian hernias occur through a defect in the linea semilunaris (Figures 6.2 and 6.3), which is a fibrous union of the rectus sheath with the aponeurosis or surgical incision. Spigelian hernias have a high frequency of incarceration.[5]

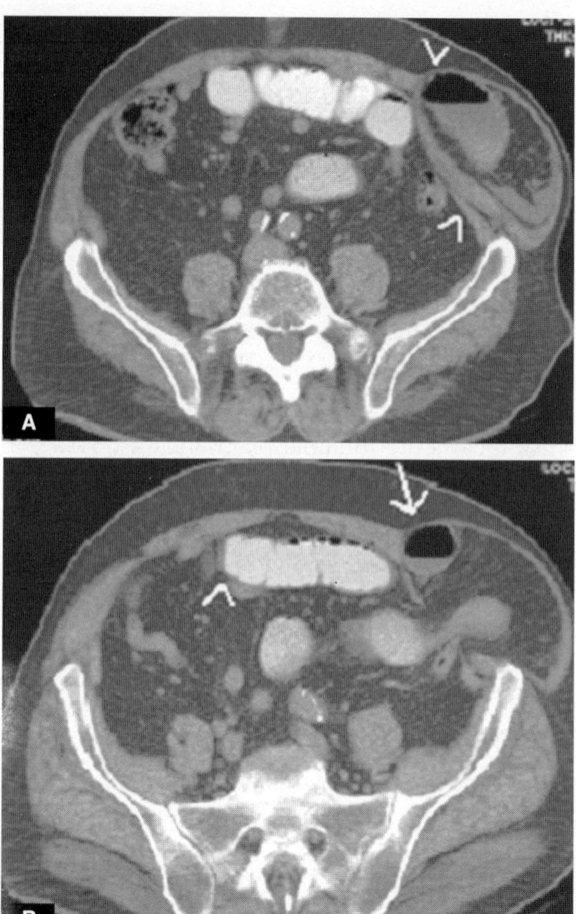

FIGURES 6.2A and B: A case of left spigelian hernia with small bowel obstruction. (A) Axial scans showing a left spigelian hernia (small arrows). (B) Axial scan slightly inferiorly showing the left spigelian hernia containing an obstructed loop within the hernia (large arrow) and dilated proximal small bowel (small arrow) with transition at the hernial site

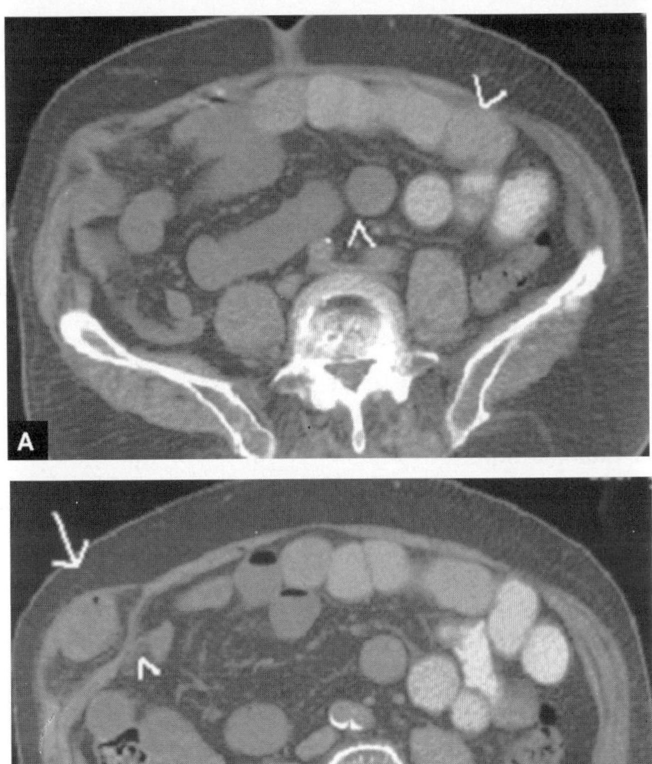

FIGURES 6.3A and B: Another example of spigelian hernia with small bowel obstruction. (A) Axial scan showing multiple dilated small bowel loops (small arrows). (B) There is a right spigelian hernia (large arrow) with transition at the site of hernia (small arrow)

Posterior Defects

Lumbar hernias occur spontaneously, post surgically or secondary to trauma. Diffuse lumbar hernias can occur after flank incision for nephrectomy. Bowel loops, retroperitoneal fat, or other visceral fat may protrude through the hernia defect. Incarceration and strangulation may occur.

INCISIONAL HERNIAS

Incisional hernias occur as delayed complications of abdominal surgery (Figure 6.4) and occur in 0.5-13.9% of patients reported series.[6]

The risk factors are obesity, postoperative wound infection, ascites, chronic pulmonary diseases, and malnutrition.

Parastomal hernias are incisional hernias. They occur adjacent to stoma and are aggravated by obesity, chronic cough or abdominal distension. CT shows bowel loops protruding through the wall defect at the stomal site (Figure 6.5).

Miscellaneous

The other hernias are less common and include Richter's hernia and obturator hernia.

In Richter's hernia, only the antimesenteric wall of the bowel is herniated (Figure 6.6). Usually the symptoms arise from strangulation and occur more frequently in femoral hernia or at the site of laparoscopic surgery.[7]

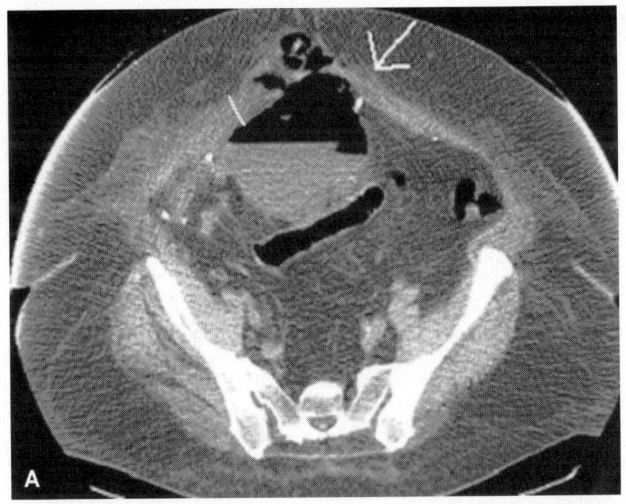

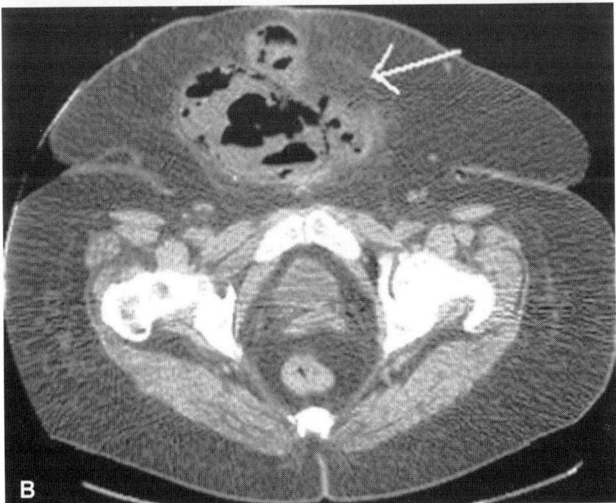

FIGURES 6.4A and B: Patient with history of prior surgery presenting with severe lower abdominal patient. (A,B) Axial scans demonstrating a lower abdominal wall hernia containing stranulated bowel (arrows)

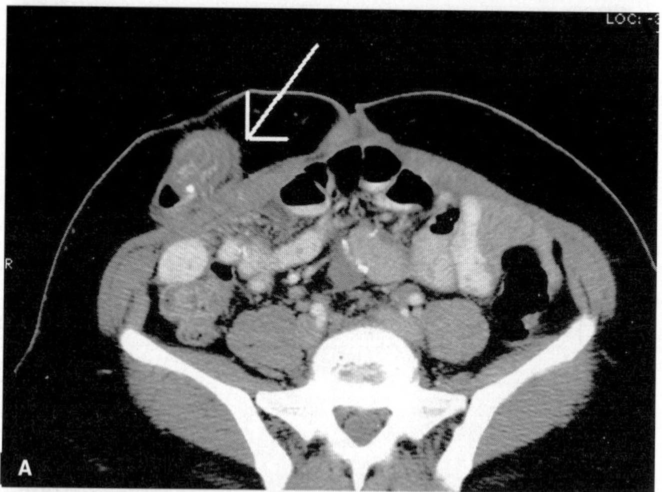

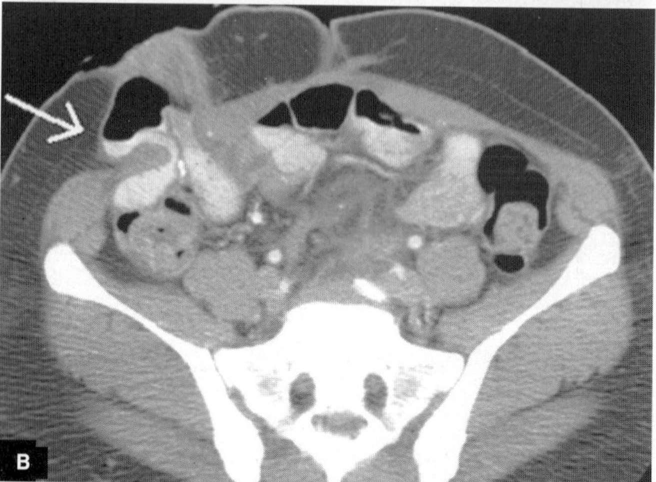

FIGURES 6.5A and B: An example of parastomal hernia. (A) Axial scan showing a right lower quadrant ileostomy (arrow). (B) Note the herniation of contrast filled distal small bowel (arrow) at the site of the stoma

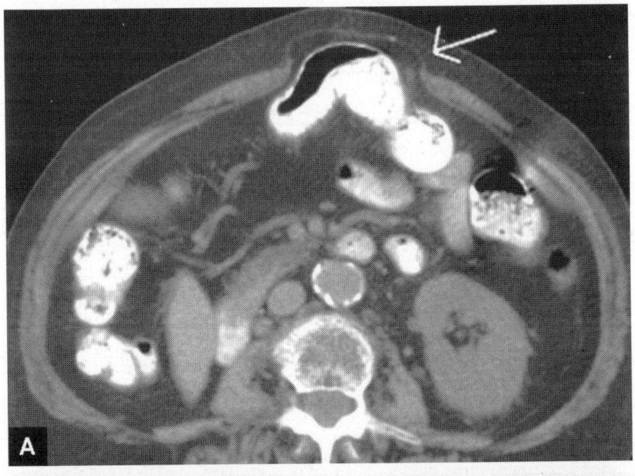

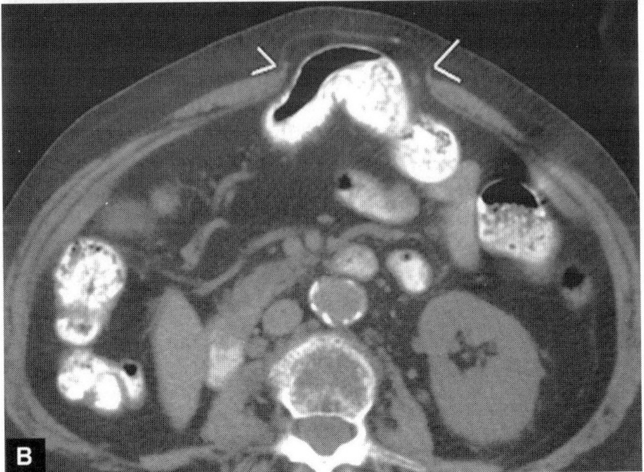

FIGURES 6.6A and B: Patient with history of mid abdominal pain. (A) Axial scan shows a small mid line ventral abdominal hernia containing a portion of large bowel (arrow). (B) Again note is a small mid line ventral abdominal hernia containing a portion of large bowel, consistent with Ritcher's hernia. Note the defect in the rectus sheath (small arrows in figure B)

OBTURATOR HERNIA

An obturator hernia is a rare but serious condition that occurs mostly in elderly, debilitated women. Obturator hernias are up to five times more common in woman than in men and may be secondary to anatomic changes in the pelvis in elderly women or to hormonal changes.

Signs and symptoms are often nonspecific, making a preoperative diagnosis uncommon.[8] Obturator hernias have the highest mortality rate (13-40%) of all abdominal wall hernias.[9] Patients may present with signs of small bowel obstruction with cramping, abdominal pain, and vomiting. The most specific finding for an obturator hernia is pain that extends down the medial aspect of thigh on abduction, extension or internal rotation. This is known as positive "Howship -Romberg sign".[10] However, this sign is present in less than one half of the patients and presence of small bowel obstruction in any elderly debilitated woman should raise the suspicion of an obturator hernia.

CT scan is the study of choice in diagnosing an obturator hernia. Obturator hernia is protrusion of the peritoneal sac through the obturator foramen and lies between the pectineal and obturator muscles. On CT scan, a well defined soft tissue density or the presence of bowel between the pectineus and obturator muscles is characteristic (Figure 6.7).

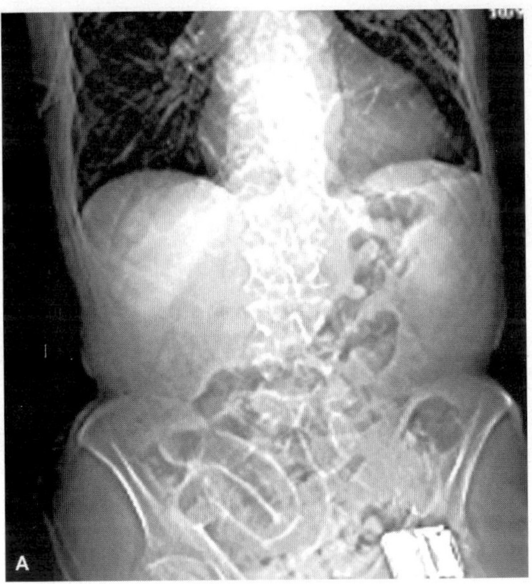

6.7A

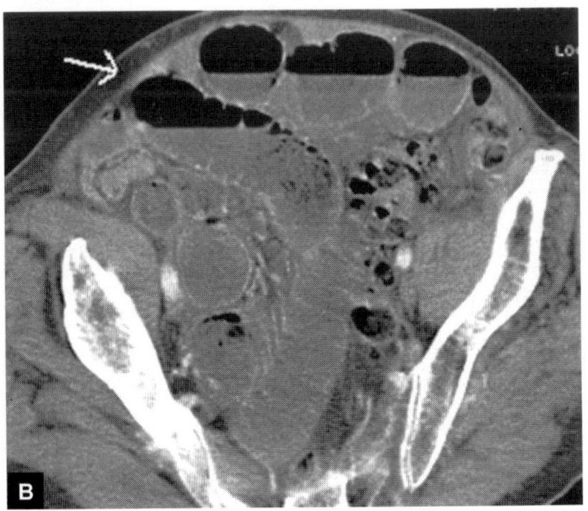

6.7B

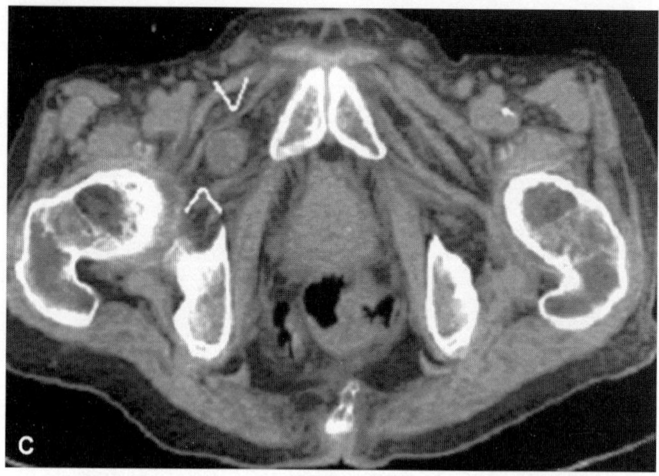

6.7C

FIGURES 6.7A to C: An elderly patient presenting with right groin pain and abdominal distension. (A) Topogram showing dilated small bowel loops in the pelvis. (B) Axial scan showing multiple dilated small bowel loops (arrow). (C) There is a rounded soft tissue density in the right obturator foramen consistent with a obturator hernia causing small bowel obstruction

CONCLUSION

Abdominal wall hernias are not uncommon. Patients may present with mild abdominal pain to severe signs of complications of hernia like incarceration, bowel obstruction, or strangulation. CT can detect the type, site and related complication. Radiologists should carefully assess the abdominal wall and detect the hernial site, size, contents and its complications.

POINTS TO REMEMBER

1. Always scan to the level of symphysis to look for groin diseases.
2. Look for signs of incarceration or strangulation.

REFERENCES

1. Herlinger H, Rubesin SE. Obstruction In: Gore RM, Levine MS, Laufer I, (Eds): Textbook of Gastrointestinal Radiology; vol I Philadelphia: Saunders, 1994; 931-66.
2. Rutkow IM. Demographic and socioeconomic aspects of hernia repair in the United States in 2003. Surg Clin North Am 2003; 83: 1045-51.
3. Harrison LA, Keesling CA, Martin NL, Lee Kr, Wetzel LH. Abdominal wall hernias review of herniography and correlation with cross-sectional imaging radiographics 1995; 15: 315-32.
4. Zarvan NP, Lee FT Jr, Yandons DR, Unger JS. Abdominal hernias: CT findings. AJR 1995; 164: 1391-95.
5. Stabile Tanora AA, Midiri M, Vince R, Rotondo A, Angelelli G. Abdominal wall hernias: Imaging with spiral CT Eur Radial 10; 914-9.
6. Ghahremani GG, Jimenez MA, Rosefield M, Rochester D. CT diagnosis of occult incisional hernias AJR 1987; 148: 139-42.
7. Mattheus BD, Heniford T, Sing RF, Preperitoneal Richter hernia after a laparoscopic gastric bypass surg laparose Endosc Percutan Tech 2001; 11: 47-9.
8. Bergstein TM, Condon RE. Obturator hernia: current diagnosis and treatment. Surgery 1996; 119: 133-6.
9. Way LW (Ed): Current Surgical Diagnosis and Treatment. 10th ed, Norwalk Conn: Appleton Lange, 1994: 712-24.
10. Schwartz ST, Ed. Principles of Surgery. 6th ed, New York: McGraw Hill, 1994: 1518-36.

CHAPTER 7

CT in Inflammatory Bowel Diseases and Infectious Colitis

INTRODUCTION

Computed tomography is increasingly being used as a technique for detection and characterization of intestinal disease because of the growing body of information that indicates that:

a. A wide spectrum of intestinal wall morphologic and enhancement abnormalities can be seen with bowel disorders.
b. CT can be used in the appropriate setting as a problem solving tool for many gastrointestinal disorders.

SCANNING TECHNIQUE

The conventional CT technique consists of scanning the abdomen after the oral and intravenous administration of contrast material. The abdomen is routinely imaged from the diaphragm to the symphysis pubis. Oral contrast typically consists of 600-900 ml of 2.5% diluted sodium amidotrizoate and meglumine amidotrizoate mixture ideally administered approximately 4 hours, 2 hours and immediately before scanning. Helical scanning with contiguous 5 mm sections is performed.

Intravenous administration of contrast material is essential, especially if extracolonic extension of disease is suspected. 100-150 ml of nonionic water soluble iodinated contrast medium is intravenously injected at a rate of 2 ml/sec through a 20 gauge intravenous catheter and scanning is performed after a 70 second delay. This delay corresponds to the portal venous phase of liver imaging.

In emergent situations or in patients in whom limited rectosigmoid disease is suspected, positive contrast agents can be administered directly into the colon via a rectum catheter.

When spiral CT is used, it is recommended that a 5 mm collimation with a table speed of 8 mm/sec be utilized. These settings correspond to a pitch of 1.6. Reconstruction of data is typically performed at 5 mm intervals.[1]

If three dimensional imaging of the colon is desired, 3 mm collimation is optimal, with a table speed of 5 mm/sec (pitch of 1.7) and 2 mm reconstruction.[1]

NORMAL COLON

The colon normally frames the abdomen and is surrounded by homogeneous fat.

The wall of the normal colon is very thin and should measure less than 3 mm.[2] When the lumen is distended, normal bowel wall thickness is 1-2 mm. When the lumen is collapsed, normal thickness may be 3-4 mm.[3] The colonic wall is barely perceptible if the colon is well distended with contrast material or air. Gas, feces and minimal fluid are normally present in the colon. Carefully following the colonic wall to a region where the colon is well distended with gas often reveals its true thickness.

CT ENHANCEMENT PATTERNS

The normal bowel wall enhances after an adequate bolus of intravenous contrast material. The enhancement is more easily identified in patients who are given water as oral contrast agent. Enhancement is usually greater on the mucosal aspect of the bowel wall. This should not be mistaken for a disease process.

Bowel wall thickening may be related to a number of entities, including normal variants, inflammatory conditions and neoplastic disease.

The attenuation pattern of a thickened segment of bowel wall is an important criteria for establishing a differential diagnosis.

Wittenberg et al describe five categories of attenuation patterns—white, grey, water halo sign, fat halo sign and black.[4]

The attenuation pattern is directly related to the administration of intravenous contrast material. Exceptions to this are the presence of central fat deposition and intestinal pneumatosis (black) . In these cases variation in attenuation of the bowel wall can be depicted on CT without intravenous contrast material because of the marked differences in tissue attenuation.

White Attenuation

This refers to the pattern of increased bowel wall enhancement seen in inflammatory bowel disease, due to hyperemic and hypervascular state seen classically with acute inflammation.[5,6] This pattern affects the majority of thickened bowel walls. A useful reference point—the bowel wall is enhanced to a degree equal to or greater than that of venous opacification in the same scan.

Mesenteric vascular dilatation and tortuosity also reflects this hypervascularity.

Caution: This pattern may also be seen in several vascular disorders.

Gray Attenuation

In this pattern the thickened bowel wall demonstrates little clear-cut enhancement and its attenuation is comparable with that of enhanced muscle. This pattern is least specific of the five categories for diagnosis and is common in both benign and malignant diseases.[4]

Water Halo Sign

Water halo sign consists of:

a. Double halo sign
b. Target sign

a. The double halo sign is composed of either
   i. an enhancing muscularis propria surrounding unenhancing submucosa and mucosa[1,5,7,8] or
   ii. an enhancing mucosa surrounded by unenhancing submucosa and muscularis propria (see Figure 7.1A)

b. The "target sign" is composed of three rings. Target sign consists of enhancement of the mucosa, and muscularis propria with interposed low attenuation edematous submucosa.[3]

   The common conditions in which this sign is seen include idiopathic inflammatory bowel disease, vascular disorders, infectious diseases and radiation damage.

Fat Halo Sign

Indicates a three-layered target sign of thickened bowel in which the middle or submucosal layer demonstrates fatty attenuation.[5,7,9,10] The detection of fat halo sign in small intestine is highly suggestive of Crohn's disease and by itself is a sign of a chronic phase.[4] It indicates ulcerative colitis or Crohn's disease when detected in the colon.

Black Attenuation

Refers to the markedly low attenuation in the bowel wall seen with pneumatosis. This pattern may be seen in ischemia as well as with infection.

Inflammatory Bowel Disease

CT has the advantage of differentiating Crohn's disease and ulcerative colitis and provide information about extraluminal disease, which is important for accurate diagnosis. Although barium studies remain the principal tool for diagnosis and evaluation of suspected inflammatory bowel disease these provide exquisite mucosal details but afford little information about extraluminal disease.

There is considerable overlap between CT findings in Crohn's disease and in ulcerative colitis. However, there are features that may help distinguish the two.

Distribution of Bowel Involvement

There is more extensive involvement of right colon and small intestine in Crohn's disease, although involvement

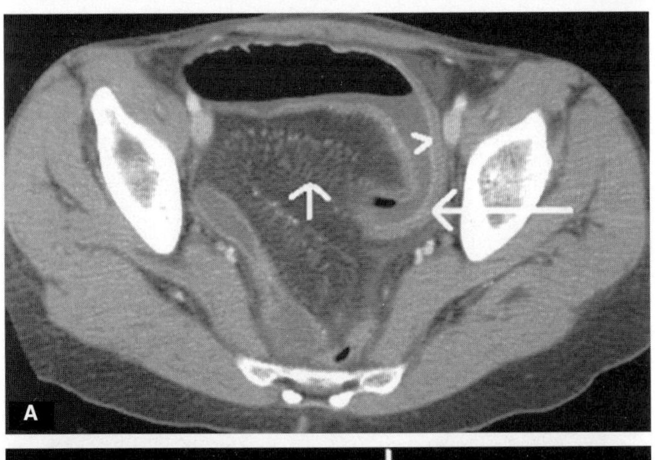

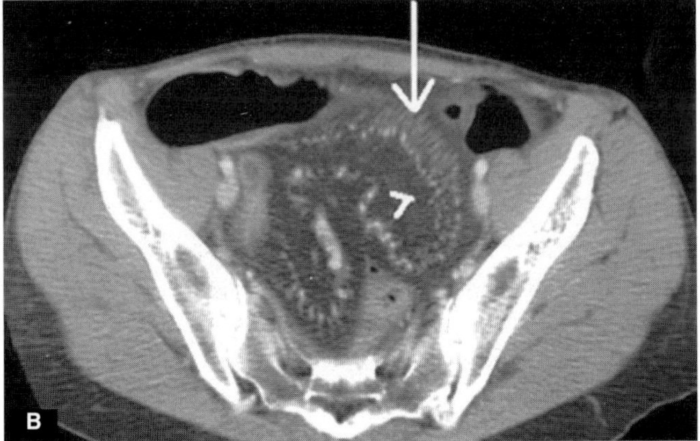

FIGURES 7.1A and B: Patient presented with abdominal pain and features suggestive of small bowel obstruction. (A) Axial scan demonstrating vascular jejunization of the ileum or the comb sign (arrow) with proliferation of the mesenteric fat-creeping fat sign (arrow head). (B) CT scan demonstrates circumferential wall thickening of the ileum with enhancement of the mucosa (arrow head), the submucosa demonstrates gray attenuation (long arrow)—Double halo sign. The CT features are consistent with Crohn's colitis with proximal small bowel loops obstruction.

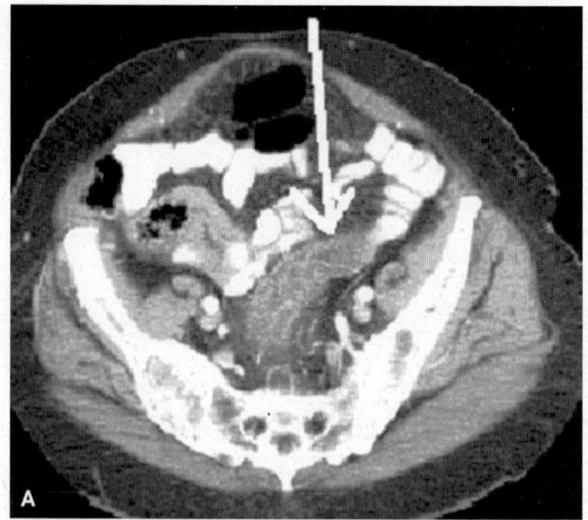

7.2A

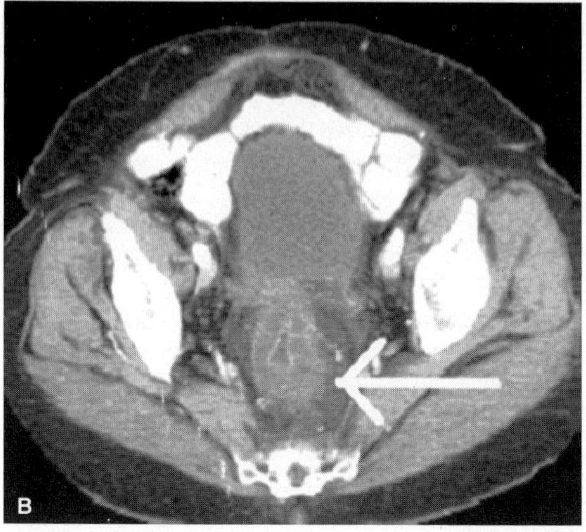

7.2B

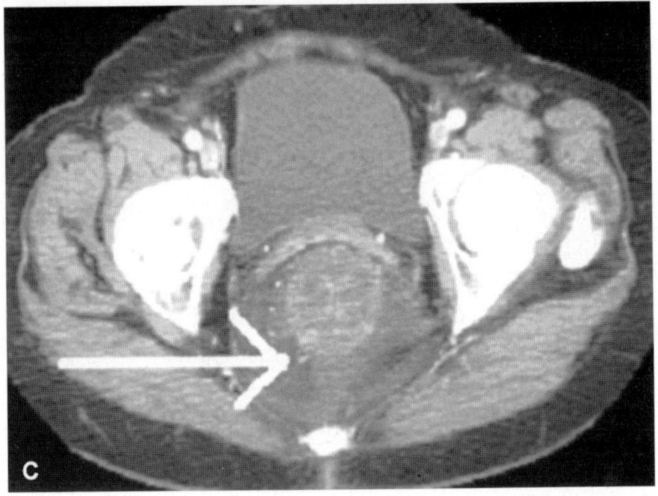

7.2C

FIGURES 7.2A to C: A case of ulcerative colitis presenting with diarrhea and pelvic pain. (A,B) Axial CT scan with oral and intravenous contrast demonstrating marked circumferential wall thickening of the sigmoid colon and rectum (arrows). (C) Caudal scan demonstrating thickened rectum with adjacent fat stranding (arrows).

of the left colon does occur. In contrast, ulcerative colitis is typically left-sided (Figure 7.2) or diffuse and only rarely involves the right colon exclusively.[9]

Bowel involvement is diffuse in ulcerative colitis, whereas it is segmental with skip regions in Crohn's disease.

Wall Thickening

At CT, the most frequent finding is wall thickening. The mean wall thickness in Crohn's disease is 11-33 mm, usually significantly greater than in ulcerative colitis (7.8 mm).[9,11] The reason for this is that the disease process is typically transmural in Crohn's disease and is limited to the mucosa in ulcerative colitis, causing greater bowel wall thickness in Crohn's disease.

Both Crohn's and ulcerative colitis demonstrate symmetrical bowel wall thickening (Figure 7.3).

Asymmetric or eccentric bowel thickening when seen, is more likely to occur in cases of long stranding Crohn's disease, which typically occurs along the mesenteric border of the intestine and can result in formation of pseudodiverticula along the antimesenteric border. Pseudodiverticula are small outpouchings of the colonic wall that occur in the stretched-thin segment of the bowel wall opposite to the regions of fibrosis and scarring.

Asymmetry is mainly seen with malignant conditions. In asymmetric bowel wall thickening of long standing Crohn's disease, the associated mesenteric findings help differentiate it from malignant conditions.[7]

Mesenteric Changes

Proliferation of mesenteric fat is an important and specific sign of Crohn's disease. However, proliferation of perirectal fat is nonspecific and can be present in, ulcerative colitis, pseudomembranous colitis or radiation colitis as well as in Crohn's disease.[9]

In Crohn's disease, there is prominence (dilatation) and separation of the vasa recta in the ileum due to increased mesenteric fat deposition ("creeping fat sign").

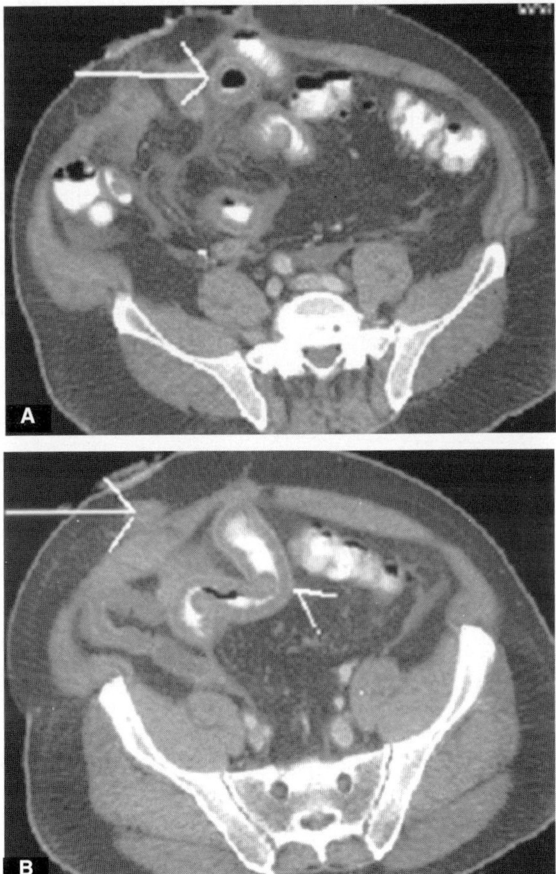

FIGURES 7.3A and B: Postoperative case of Crohn's disease presenting with abdominal pain. (A) CT scan demonstrates acute exacerbation of Crohn's disease with wall thickening of the ileum and adjacent fat stranding (arrow). (B) Postoperative changes in the anterior abdominal wall (arrow) and wall thickening of the ileum (arrow head).

This is called vascular jejunization of the ileum or "comb sign" (Figure 7.1B).[12,13]

Fibrofatty proliferation of the mesentery is the primary cause of bowel displacement in Crohn's disease however, lymphadenopathy is the cause in Tuberculosis.[14] This helps in differentiating the two. In the setting of inflammatory bowel disease, mesenteric lymphadenopathy suggests Crohn's disease rather than ulcerative colitis, although in general it is not a specific finding for inflammatory bowel disease.

Bowel Wall Attenuation Pattern

Heterogeneous (stratified) attenuation pattern may be seen in the form of Double halo and target sign.

The findings of stratified attenuation, although nonspecific is used mainly to exclude malignant condition.[7]

Inflammed mucosa and serosa may enhance markedly after intravenous administration of iodinated contrast and the intensity of enhancement correlates with the clinical activity of the disease.[15]

The observation of fat halo sign (target sign) in the small intestine is highly suggestive of Crohn's disease and by itself is a sign of chronic phase. Both acute and chronic disease patterns may coexist in the same patient, ie the fat halo and water halo signs may both be seen in a patient in different segments of the bowel.[5]

The fat halo sign, when seen in the colon may indicate either ulcerative colitis or Crohn's disease.[5] One study found submucosal fat deposition in the colon in 61% of patients with ulcerative colitis but in only 8% of patients with Crohn's disease[9] indicating that fat halo sign is more common in ulcerative colitis.[9]

In general, fat deposition in the bowel wall indicates inactive disease in both Crohn's disease and ulcerative colitis.

Complications of Inflammatory Bowel Disease

Abscesses are typically seen in Crohn's disease (Figure7.4) and not in ulcerative colitis.[9, 16] An abscess can be confined to the bowel wall and pericolic fat or can involve bladder, psoas muscle, and the pelvic sidewall. Fistulas are a common secondary finding in Crohn's disease and aid in its diagnosis. Enterovesical, enterocutaneous, perianal and rectovaginal fistulas can all be detected with CT.

In suspected enterovesical fistula, CT is performed with oral or rectal contrast material without intravenous contrast to avoid contrast excretion into the urinary bladder.

In the advanced ,stenotic phase of Crohn's disease, patients frequently present with recurrent episodes of partial small bowel obstruction.High grade obstructions are rare.[15]

Typhlitis

Also known as neutropenic enterocolitis.

It is commonly seen in patients with acute leukemia under chemotherapy who have severe neutropenia. The condition is characterized by inflammation and edema of the cecum, ascending colon and rarely terminal ileum.

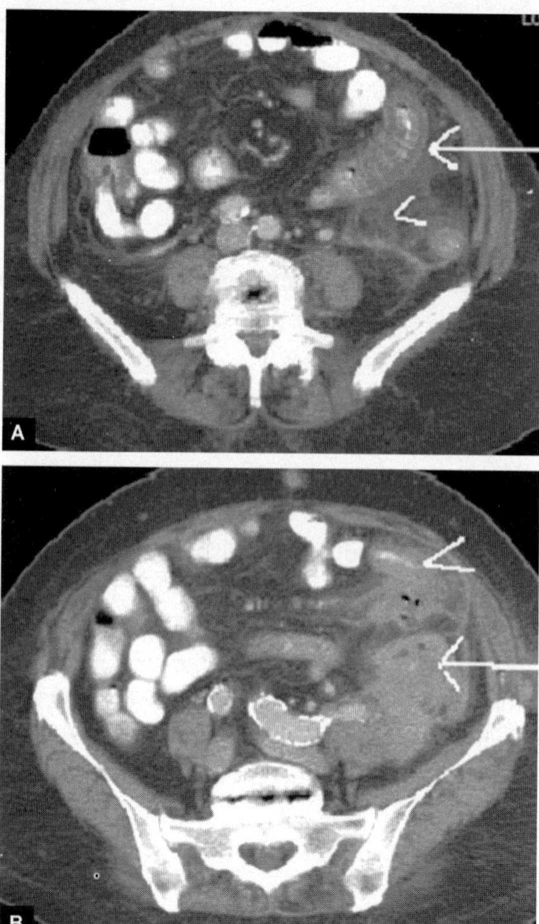

FIGURES 7.4A and B: A known patient of Crohn's disease presented with abdominal pain and fever. (A) CT scan demonstrates marked wall thickening of the ileum (arrow) with extensive adjacent fat stranding (arrow head). (B) Caudal CT sections demonstrate fluid collections with loculi of air suggestive of abscesses (arrow)—complication of Crohn's disease.

The patient presents with fever, watery diarrhea and abdominal pain localized to the right lower quadrant. A combination of various mechanisms like ischemia, infection (especially with Cytomegalovirus) , mucosal hemorrhage and neoplastic infiltration,[17] may be the cause for the inflammation, as the precise cause is not known. Complications like transmural necrosis, perforation and death can result. Treatment consists of bowel rest, total parenteral nutrition, antibiotics, aggressive fluid and electrolyte replacement.

CT is suggested for diagnosis of typhlitis as colonoscopy or contrast enema examination increases the risk of bowel perforation. CT demonstrates cecal distention and circumferential thickening of the cecal wall (Figure 7.5).

Adjacent mesenteric fat demonstrating inflammatory stranding is a common finding. Complications such as pneumatosis, pneumoperitoneum and pericolic fluid collection need to be detected at the earliest because they indicate a need for urgent surgical management.[18,19] It may be difficult to differentiate typhilitis from appendicitis or Crohn's disease on the basis of CT findings alone owing to the involvement of cecum. Clinical presentation and history, which are distinctive, must be correlated with CT findings.

Radiation Colitis

Radiation therapy can cause acute radiation injury to the small intestine and colon within a few weeks of radiation exposure. Patients present with self-limited diarrhoea.

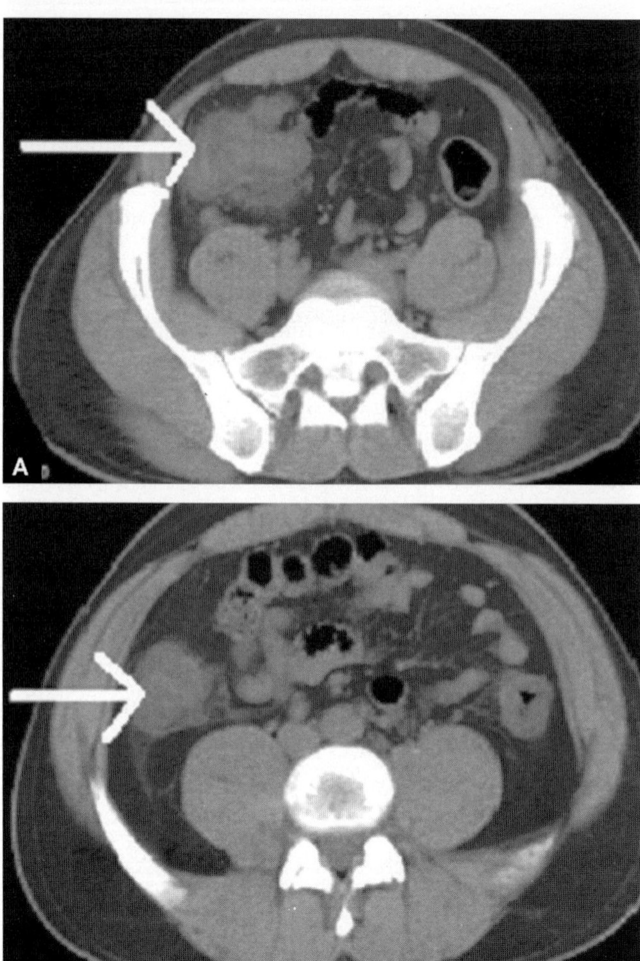

FIGURES 7.5A and B: Patient of leukemia under chemotherapy with severe neutropenia presented with fever, watery diarrhoea and fever. (A,B) CT scan demonstrates circumferential thickening of the cecal wall (arrows) with adjacent fat stranding suggestive of typhlitis.

If CT is performed in such patients, nonspecific wall thickening and inflammatory stranding will be demonstrated in the affected region, which is typically the rectosigmoid in patients who have undergone pelvic radiation for prostate or cervical cancer.

Over one half of patients receiving greater than 3000 cGy of radiation to the pelvis develop acute proctitis which manifest as pain, diarrhoea, tenesmus and rectal bleeding.[20] Proctitis is self-limited and is treated symptomatically.

Acute radiation injury is usually detected clinically and treated conservatively. Imaging is typically not necessary for diagnosis.

Chronic radiation injury of the colon and rectum can occur with the majority of patients presenting 6-24 months after completion of radiation therapy.[21] Since radiation therapy is often given for pelvic disease, the sigmoid colon and rectum are the most commonly affected and in this case colitis represents the result of radiation induced arteritis.[9]

Chronic radiation enteritis may show homogeneous attenuation on contrast enhanced CT.[5, 22] Nonspecific wall thickening typically in the rectum is seen; increased pelvic fat and thickening of perirectal fibrous tissue are also seen.[23] Strictures and fistulas are possible complications. Since the CT findings are nonspecific, clinical history is the key to diagnosis.

Pseudomembranous Colitis

Pseudomembranous colitis is caused by toxins produced by an overgrowth of the organism Clostridium difficile, resulting in profuse watery diarrhoea, abdominal pain and fever.[24]

This condition was first described as a complication of antibiotic therapy, but was also found to be associated with hypotensive episodes, chemotherapeutic agents and abdominal surgery. The diagnosis is typically made with stool assay for the Clostridium difficile toxin.

CT findings are important because the clinical findings are often nonspecific and the diagnosis may therefore not be suspected. If not treated aggressively, pseudomembranous colitis results in significant morbidity and mortality.[25, 26] Treatment with metronidazole and vancomycin is usually effective.

The most common (but nonspecific) CT finding in pseudomembranous colitis is thickening of the colonic wall, circumferential or eccentric.

One series showed colonic wall thickness ranging from 3 to 32 mm (mean 14.7 mm).[27] Another series showed mean colonic wall thickness of 10.7 mm.[9] In general, the bowel wall thickening in pseudomembranous colitis is greater than in any other inflammatory or infectious disease of the colon except Crohn's disease; this is a helpful differentiating point.[28] In pseudomembranous colitis the wall thickening is irregular and shaggy, whereas in Crohn's disease, it is symmetric and homogeneous.[27]

Mild pericolic stranding may be present. Although a nonspecific finding occurring in other inflammatory and infectious colonic diseases, the pericolic stranding in pseudomembranous colitis is often disproportionately mild relative to the marked colonic wall thickening, since the condition predominantly affects mucosa and submucosa.[29] When haustral folds are thickened, they appear as broad transverse bands that may trap oral contrast material (Figure 7.6) . This appearance is known as the accordion sign.[27] This is a very suggestive feature of the disease but typically occurs only in severe cases and is therefore not a sensitive indicator.

Classically, pseudomembranous colitis is a pancolitis. However, in some cases it can be limited to the right side of the colon sparing the left colon in up to 30-40% of cases.[28] Isolated segments of the colon and rectum can be involved.[27, 28]

Ascites is reported in up to 35% of patients, both as a direct complication of the infection and due to co-existing conditions such as portal hypertension.[28, 30] Thus, ascites is helpful in differentiating pseudomembranous colitis from Crohn's colitis. However, ascites is not uncommon in infectious colitis and ischemia.

Infectious Colitis

Infectious colitis is caused by various organisms.

Bacterial causes include Shigella, Salmonella, Yersenia, Campylobacter, Staphylococcus and Chlamydia trachomatis.

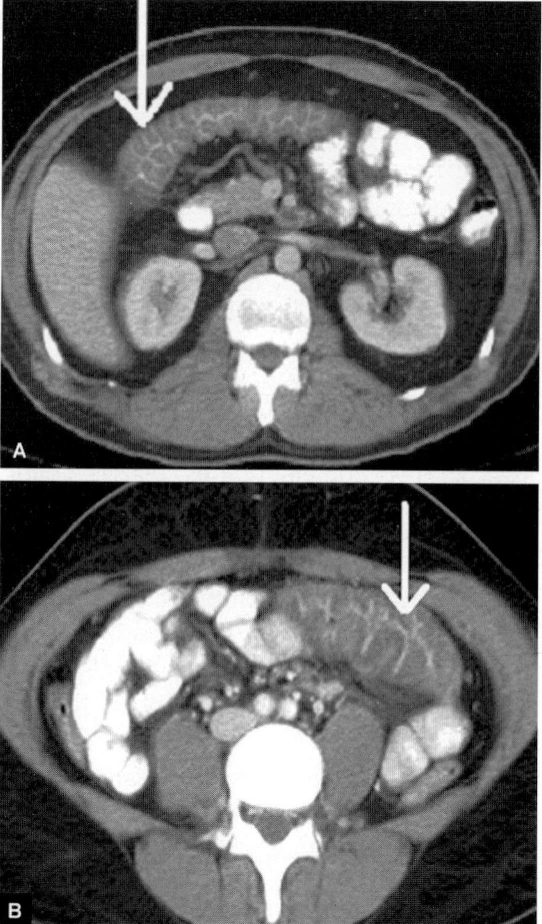

FIGURES 7.6A and B: Patient who was on antibiotic therapy presented with abdominal pain, profuse watery diarrhoea and fever. (A,B) CT scan demonstrates marked thickening of the haustral folds in the transverse colon with trapped oral contrast material (arrows)—this appearance is known as accordion sign suggestive of Pseudomembranous colitis.

Fungal infections include histoplasmosis, mucormycosis and actinomycosis.

Viral causes include herpesvirus, Cytomegalovirus and rotavirus.

Ameobiasis and tuberculosis can also cause colitis, which can resemble inflammatory bowel disease.

Infectious colitides are typically diagnosed clinically and do not require CT.

At CT, patients with infectious colitis from any cause typically have wall thickening, which demonstrates homogeneous enhancement.

Ascites or inflammation of the pericolic fat may also be present.[9] Multiple air fluid levels may be present in the colon due to increased fluid and fluid feces. The portion of colon affected may suggest a specific organism. For instance, most cases of infectious colitis are limited to the right colon (Shigella, Salmonella) , although diffuse involvement also occurs (Cytomegalovirus, E.coli).[17] In contrast, gonorrhoea, herpesvirus and chlamydia trachomatis (lymphogranuloma venereum) typically involve the rectosigmoid.

In schistosomiasis, involvement is usually confined to the descending and sigmoid colon because the adult worms have a tendency to enter the inferior mesenteric vein.

REFERENCES

1. Horton KM, Corl FM, Fishman EK. CT evaluation of the colon; inflammatory disease. Radiographics 2000; 20:399-418.

2. Fisher JK. Abnormal colonic wall thickening on computed tomography. J Comput Assist Tomogr 1983;7:90-97.
3. Balthazar EJ. CT of the gastrointestinal tract; principles and interpretation. Am J Roentgenol 1991; 156:23-32.
4. Wittenberg J et al. Algorithmic approach to CT Diagnosis of the abnormal bowel wall. Radiographics 2002; 22:1093-1109.
5. Gore RM, Balthazar EJ, Ghahremani GG, Miller FH. CT features of ulcerative colitis and Crohn's disease. Am J Roentgenol 1996; 167:3-15.
6. Tomei E, Diacinti D, Marini M, Boirivant M, Paoluzi P. Computed tomography of bowel wall in patients with Crohn's disease: relationship of inflammatory activity to biological indices. Ital J Gastroenterol 1996; 28:487-92.
7. Macari M, Balthazar EJ. CT of bowel wall thickening; significance and pitfalls of interpretation. Am J Roentgenol 2001;176(5) :1105-16.
8. Frager DH, Goldman M, Beneventano TC. Computed tomography in Crohn's disease. J Comput Assist Tomogr 1983; 7:819-24.
9. Philpotts LE, Heiken JP, Westcott MA, Gore RM. Colitis: Use of CT findings in differential diagnosis Radiology 1994; 190:445-9.
10. Jones B, Fishman EK, Hamilton SR, et al. Submucosal accumulation of fat in inflammatory bowel disease: CT/ pathologic correlation. J comput assist Tomogr 1986; 10:759-63.
11. Fishman EK, Wolf EJ, Jones B, Bayless TM, Seigelman SS, CT evaluation of Crohn's disease: Effect on patient management. AJR Am J Roentgenol 1987; 148: 537-540.
12. Meyers MA, McGuire PV. Spiral CT demonstration of hypervascularity in Crohn's disease; "vascular jejunization of the ileum" or the comb sign. Abdom Imaging 1995; 20:327-32.
13. Gore RM. CT of inflammatory bowel disease. Radiol Clin North Am 1989; 27:717-29.
14. Makanjuola D. Is it Crohn's disease or intestinal tuberculosis? CT analysis. Eur J Radiol 1998; 1:55-61.

15. Boudiaf M et al. CT evaluation of small bowel obstruction. Radiographics 2001;21:613-24.
16. Gore RM, Marn CS, Kirby DF, Vogelzang RL, Neiman HL. CT findings in ulcerative granulomatous and indeterminate colitis. AJR Am J Roentgenol 1984; 143:279-84.
17. Wall SD, Jones B. Gastrointestinal tract in the immunocompromised host; opportunistic infections and other complications. Radiology 1992; 185; 327-35.
18. Shamberger RC, Weinstein HJ, Delorey MJ, Levey RM. The medical and surgical management of typhlitis in children with acute nonlymphocytic (myelogenous) leukemia cancer 1986; 57:603-9.
19. Frick MP, Maile CW, Crass JR, Goldberg ME, Delaney JP. Computed tomography of neutropenic colitis AJR Am J Roentgenol 1984; 143; 763-5.
20. Otchy DP, Nelson H. Radiation injuries of the colon and rectum. Surg Clin North Am 1993; 73: 1017-1035.
21. Gilinsky NH, Burns DG, Barbezat GO, Levin W, Myers HS, Marks IN. The natural history of radiation induced proctosigmoiditis ; an analysis of 88 patients. QJ Med 1983; 52:40-53.
22. Rha SE, HaHK, Lee SH, et al. CT and MRI imaging features of bowel ischemia from various primary causes. Radiographics 2000, 20:29-42.
23. Frommhold W, Hutener KH. The role of computer tomography in the after care of patients suffering from carcinoma of the rectum. J Comput Assist Tomogr 1981; 5:161-8.
24. Kelly CP, Pothoulakia C, LaMont JT. *Clostridium difficile* colitis. N Engl J Med 1994; 330:257-62.
25. Jobe BA, Grasley A, Deveney KE, Deveney CW, Sheppard BC. Clostridium difficile colitis; an increasing hospital – acquired illness. Am J Surg 1995; 169: 480-83.
26. Morris JB, Zollinger RM Jr, Stellato TA. Role of surgery in antibiotic – induced pseudomembranous enterocolitis. Am J Surg 1990; 160; 535-9.

27. Fishman EK, Kavuru M, Jones B, et al. Pseudomembranous colitis; CT evaluation of 26 cases. Radiology 1991; 180; 57-60.
28. Ros PR, Buetow PC, Pantogoag–Brown L, Forsmark CE, Sobin LH. Pseudomembranous colitis. Radiology 1996; 198:1-9.
29. Merino D, Fishman EK, Jones B. Pseudomembranous colitis; CT evaluation. J comput Assist Tomogr 1987; 11:1017-20.
30. Jafri SF, Marshall LB. Ascites associated with antibiotic-associated pseudomembranous colitis. South Med J 1996; 89: 1014-17.

CHAPTER 8

Ischemic Bowel Disease

INTRODUCTION

Bowel ischemia is a process of insufficient blood supply to the small or large bowel with consequences ranging from a transient reversible condition to a lethal catastrophic event.

Bowel ischemia is caused by various conditions. It may result directly from:

a. Arterial occlusion, e.g. Occlusion of SMA, vasculitis, external compression of artery by adhesions, volvulus and hernia etc.
b. Hypotension (Congestive heart failure, hypovolemia, sepsis).
c. Vasoconstrictive drugs (digitalis, norepinephrine, ergotamine).
d. Impaired venous drainage (thrombosis of SMV, portal veins, compression of the mesenteric veins by tumor, adhesions, volvulus etc) . Patients with hypercoagulable states and women on oral contraceptives are at risk.

The clinical presentation includes abdominal pain out of proportion to physical signs, nausea, vomiting, and bloody diarrhea.[1,2]

The clinical presentation varies and depends on the severity of the process, the degree of collateral vascular occlusion, arterial or venous involvement. However clinically symptoms may be nonspecific and often result in delay in diagnosis resulting in complications and mortality.

CT scan is proven to be helpful in establishing the diagnosis of bowel ischemia.[2]

PATHOPHYSIOLOGY

The severity depends on the acuteness, duration, degree and presence of collateral circulation. The damage starts with the mucosa, which is most vulnerable to ischemia and extents outward through the submucosa and the muscular layer and ends at the serosa.

CT PROTOCOL

Accurate CT imaging of acute bowel ischemia usually requires both oral and rectal administration of contrast material or water, as well as intravenous administration of iodinated contrast material. In cases where acute bowel ischemia and ischemic colitis are suspected, oral administration of 600-750 mL of contrast material or water 30-120 minutes before scanning or rectal administration of 400-800 mL of contrast material or water is important to achieve adequate bowel distension. Rectal administration of water or contrast material is especially important in cases where acute colonic ischemia is suspected, since it may otherwise be impossible, when colonic segments are contracted, to decide whether bowel wall thickening is present or the CT findings only represent colonic contraction.

Intravenous administration of contrast material is necessary to demonstrate the presence of thrombi in the mesenteric arteries or veins, although additional acquisition of unenhanced CT scans may help delineate vascular calcifications, hyperattenuating intravascular clotting, and acute submucosal or intramural hemorrhage

About 100 to 150 mL of contrast material (300-370 mg of iodine per milliliter) is usually administered with a power injector at a rate of 2-4 mL/sec

Acquisition of arterial phase CT scans and CT angiograms is of great value in the assessment of mesenteric arteries.

However, high-quality portal venous phase scans are usually sufficient to show occlusions of mesenteric arteries and have the additional advantages of

i. Depicting mesenteric veins;
ii. Allowing better assessment of abnormalities of the bowel wall itself; and
iii. Providing greater accuracy in the detection of perforation, abscess formation, and peritonitis, as well as in the diagnosis of other causes of acute abdomen.

CT FINDINGS IN BOWEL ISCHEMIA

The CT findings evolve as the process in the bowel wall progresses from ischemia to infarction.

Early findings include mural thickening of the involved segment usually related to intramural edema. As the process progresses, there may be intramural hemorrhages. Some amount of stranding and haziness can be seen in the adjacent mesentery. During the early stages of ischemia, a target sign can be identified in the bowel wall, related to intramural edema.[3] As the process of ischemia progresses further, there may be decreased attenuation and enhancement of the affected bowel wall and the intestinal wall may become thin.[3, 4]

The early CT findings of bowel ischemia including bowel wall thickening, target sign and mesenteric stranding are not specific to bowel ischemia. They can also be seen in various inflammatory or infectious bowel pathologies, in radiation changes and very often in intramural hemorrhage.

In the later stage of continued ischemia and infarction, there may be bacterial proliferation and gas production. This gas may dissect into the necrotic wall (pneumatosis intestinalis) (Figure 8.1), spread to the mesenteric veins and finally flow into the portal veins (Figure 8.2).

Evaluation of the SMA, and SMV can show presence of occlusion or thrombosis. CT is useful in detecting an occluded or thrombosed SMV or SMA (Figure 8.3).

Thus given the presence of pneumatosis, thrombus in the SMA or SMV along with air in the mesenteric and the portal veins, a specific diagnosis can be made. The presence of air in the bowel wall, mesentery and portal venous system has grave prognostic implications in bowel ischemia. CT is more sensitive than plain film in detecting pneumatosis and portal venous gas.[5-7]

Other associated secondary findings like a small caliber aorta and SMA or a collapsed IVC may suggest hypotensive shock and low flow non-occlusive ischemia.

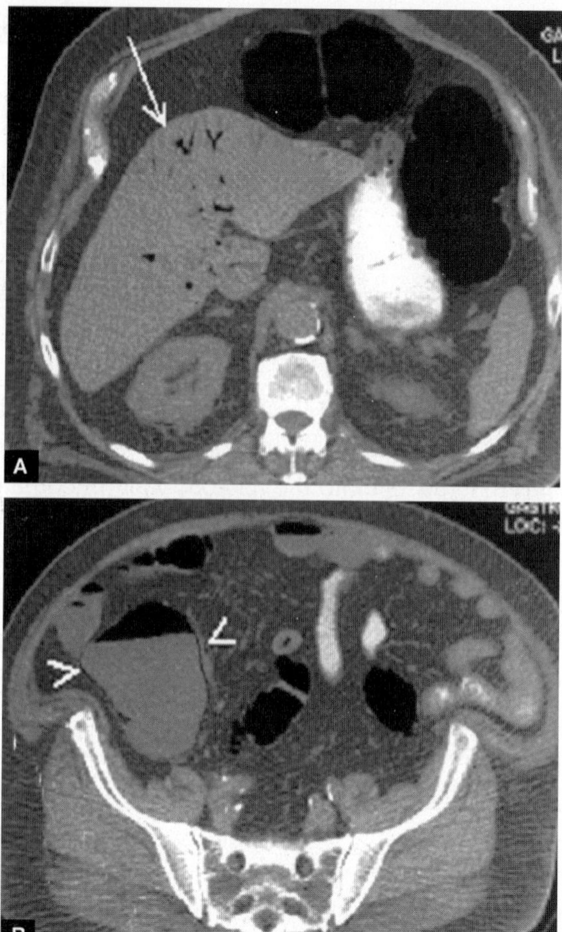

FIGURES 8.1A and B: Patient presenting with abdominal pain and bloody diarrhea. (A) Non-contrast scan showing air within the intrahepatic portal venous radicals (arrow). (B) Inferior scans showing dilated cecum with pneumatosis (small arrows) consistent with ischemic colitis

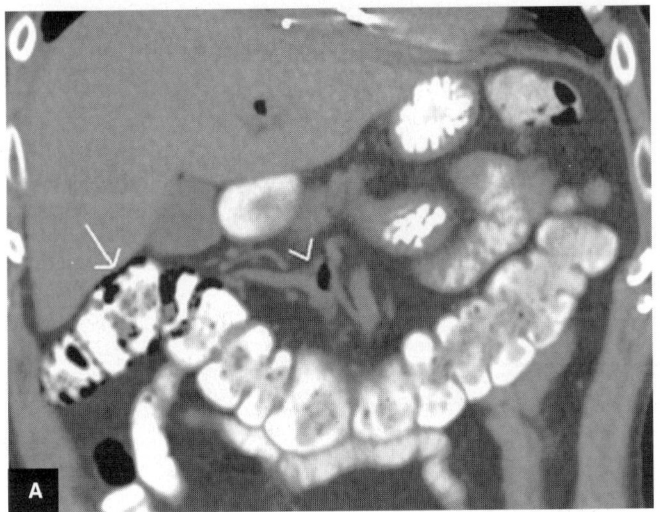

8.2A

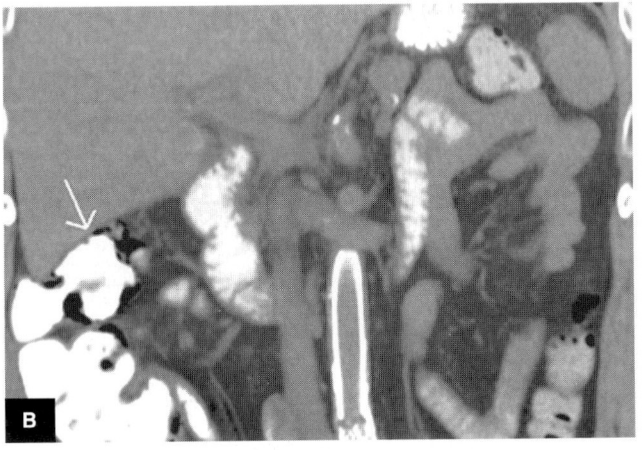

8.2B

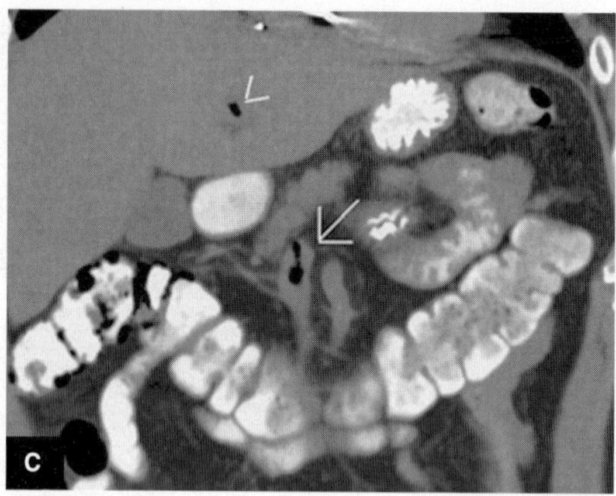

8.2C

FIGURES 8.2A to C: Patient presented with acute abdominal pain and bloody diarrhea and suspected colitis. (A,B) Coronal reformat images with oral and rectal contrast demonstrating pneumatosis, air in the bowel wall in the ascending and proximal transverse colon (large arrows in Figures A and B). (C) Note there is air within the mesenteric vein (large arrow) and in the portal venous radical (small arrow) consistent with ischemic colitis

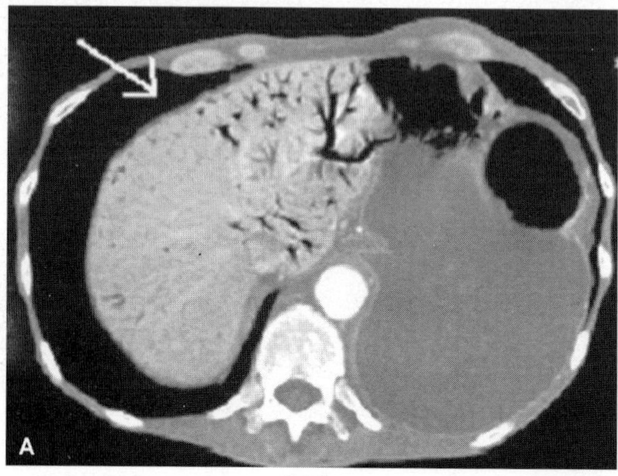

8.3A

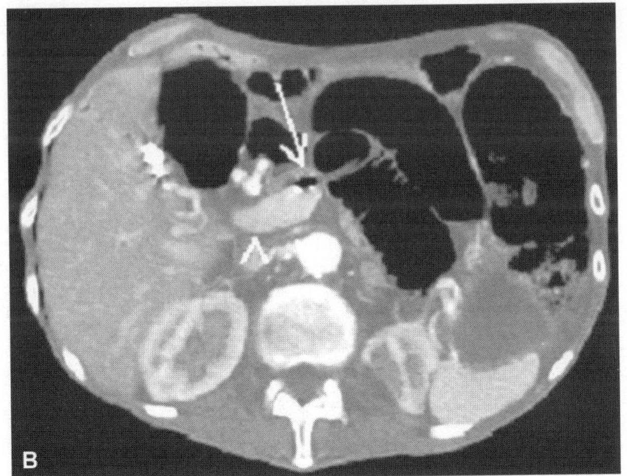

8.3B

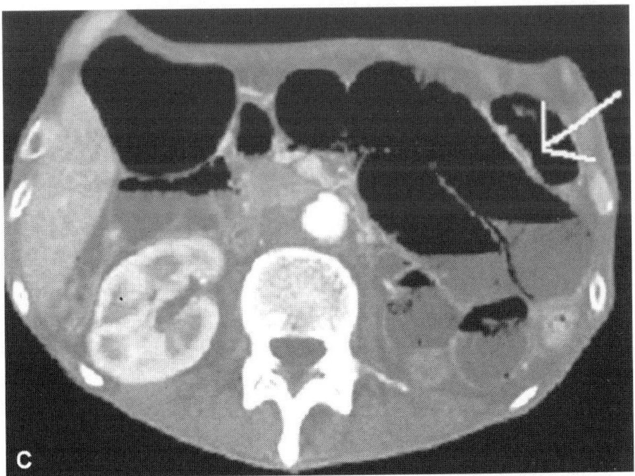

8.3C

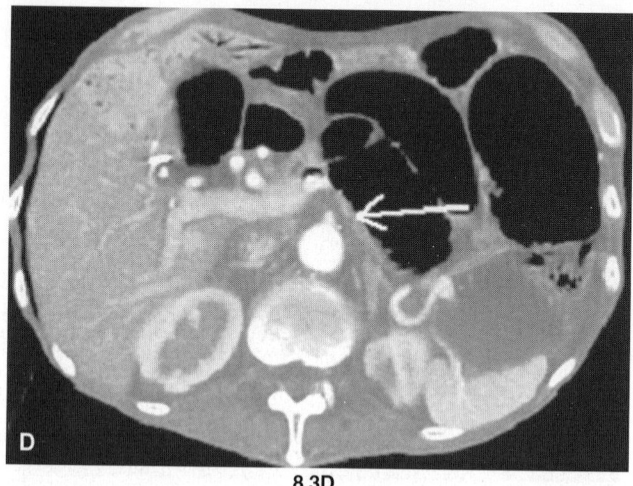

8.3D

FIGURES 8.3A to D: An elderly patient presenting with acute abdominal pain and hypotension. (A,B) Axial scans with intravenous contrast showing extensive air within the intrahepatic portal venous radicals (arrow Fig. A) and in the main portal vein (arrow Fig. B). (C) Caudal scans demonstrating fluid filled small bowel with pneumatosis (arrow). (D) Scan at the level of SMA showing abrupt cut of SMA, representing acute arterial occlusion and resultant mesenteric ischemia

Frequently on CT, intramural hemorrhage(Figure 8.4) can have identical findings of bowel wall ischemia , such as bowel wall thickening, target appearance and mesenteric stranding.

In the absence of pneumatosis or specific signs, the diagnosis may be difficult, however the presence of:

a. Short segment involvement,
b. Bowel wall thickening greater than 1 cm favor intramural hemorrhage.[8,9]

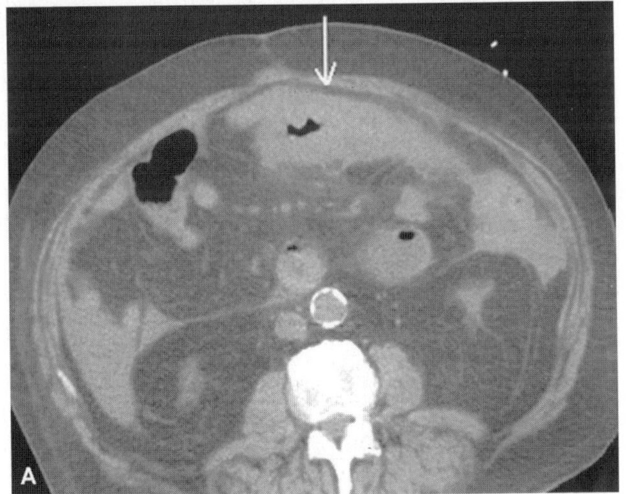

8.4A

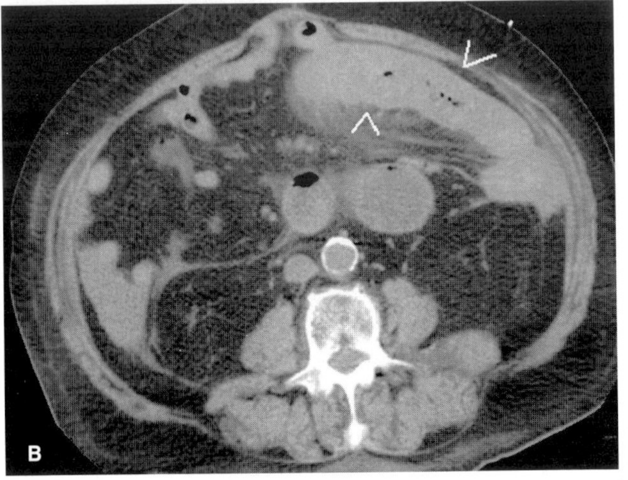

8.4B

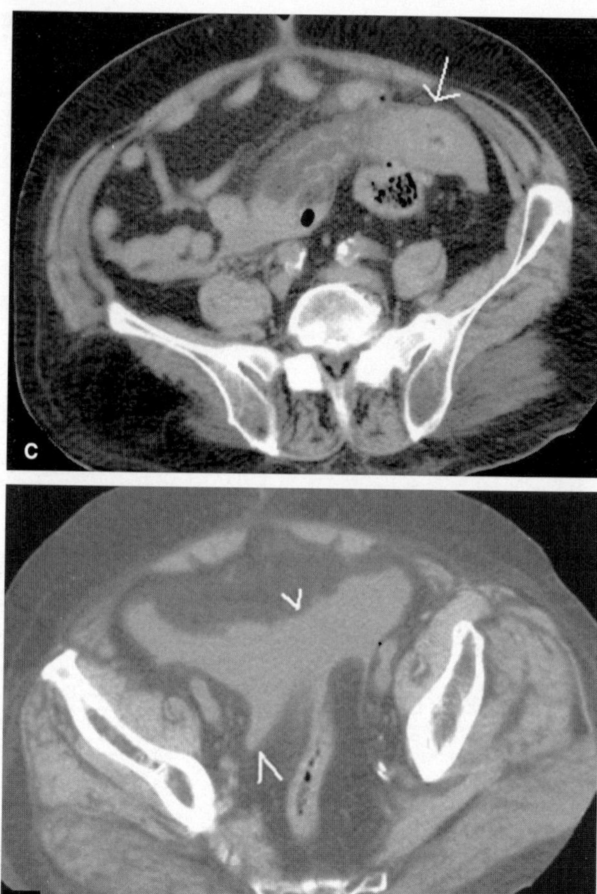

FIGURES 8.4A to D: Patient with history of anticoagulant therapy and severe abdominal pain and, suspected mesenteric ischemia. (A,B,C) Axial scans without intravenous contrast demonstrating markedly thickened small bowel loops with surrounding mesenteric stranding (arrows). (D) Hyperdense free fluid is seen in the pelvis, features consistent with intramural hemorrhage and hemoperitoneum.

Finally evaluation of the SMA and SMV is important and demonstration of occlusion or thrombus may be helpful.

In conclusion, bowel ischemia is a difficult clinical diagnosis, resulting in increased morbidity and mortality. CT is effective in detecting the early signs and makes a specific diagnosis and initiate appropriate treatment. The various CT findings described above helps in the early diagnosis.

POINTS TO REMEMBER

1. Always look for presence of portal venous gas in suspected ischemia
2. Evaluate the SMA/SMV carefully.
3. Identify the presence of abnormal bowel, look for target sign and subtle enhancement differences between the normal and abnormal bowel.

REFERENCES

1. Bartnicke BJ, Balfe DM. CT appearance of intestinal ischemia and intramural hemorrhage. Radio Clin North Am 1994; 5: 845-60.
2. Kumar S, Sarr MG, Kamath PS. Current concepts : mesenteric venous thrombosis N. Engl. JMed 2001; 345: 1683-8.
3. Rha SE, Ha HK, Lee SH, et al. CT and MR imaging findings of bowel ischemia from various primary causes. Radiographics 2000; 20: 29-42.
4. Zaleman M, Van Gansbeke D, Lalmand B, Braude P. Closet J, Strayven J. Delayed enhancement of the bowel wall : a new CT sign of small bowel strangulation J Comput Assist Tomogr 1996; 20: 379-81.

5. Levine JS, Jacobson ED. Intestinal ischemic disorders Dig: Dis 1995; 13: 3-24.
6. Smerud MJ, Johnson CD, Stephens DH. Diagnosis of bowel infarction: a comparison of plain films and CT scan in 23 cases. AJR 1990; 154: 99-103.
7. Balthazar EJ. Yen BC, Gordon RB. Ischemic colitis. CT evaluation of 54 cases. Radiology 1999; 211: 381-388.
8. Bartnicke BJ, Balfe DM. CT appearances of intestinal ischemia and intramural hemorrhage .Radiol Clin.North Am 1995; 5: 845-60
9. Michael Macari , Hersch Chandarana, Emil Balthazar,James Babb. Intestinal ischemia versus Intramural hemorrhage :CT evaluation. AJR 2003; 180: 177-184

CHAPTER 9

Acute Intra-abdominal Vascular Emergencies and Hemorrhage

INTRODUCTION

Acute intra-abdominal vascular emergencies and hemorrhage constitute an important group of acute abdomen. They range from self-limiting spontaneous hemorrhages to life-threatening ruptured abdominal aortic aneurysm. Noninvasive diagnosis is essential for confirmation and initiating early treatment to reduce morbidity and mortality. In this chapter, we will cover the CT imaging findings of common acute intra-abdominal vascular disorders and hemorrhage.

RUPTURED ABDOMINAL AORTIC ANEURYSM

Aneurysmal dilation of the abdominal aorta is defined as a diameter of more than 3 cm. Rupture of abdominal aortic aneurysm is a catastrophic complication with mortality rates approaching 95%. Up to 40% of patients die within 1 hour of the onset of symptoms.[1]

In autopsy, studies reported by Lederte et al,[2] the 1 year incidence of abdominal aortic aneurysm rupture according to initial diameter was 9.4% for diameter of 5.5-5.9 cm, 10.2% for diameters of 6.0-6.9 cm, 19.1% for the subgroup of 6.5-6.9, and 32.5% for diameters of 7.0 cm or more.

The clinical triad of symptoms of ruptured aortic aneurysms includes abdominal pain, a pulsatile mass and hypotension. Nearly a third of patients do not have the classic presentation and are misdiagnosed as having renal colic and diverticulitis. CT scan is the modality of choice for evaluation of suspected abdominal aneurysm rupture. Helical CT with quality Multiplanar and 3D images has essentially replaced conventional angiography in the evaluation of aortic aneurysm.[3]

CT TECHNIQUE AND PROTOCOL

Unenhanced images are initially obtained to search for hyperdense blood and signs of impending rupture (see below). Rapid infusion of contrast material (> 3ml/s) and thin collimation (3 mm) are required for optimal vascular resolution.[3] Oral contrast is not administered because it may interfere with CT angiographic reconstruction. Helical CT can accurately measure the diameter of the aneurysm and allow direct visualization of mural thrombus and outer aneurysm wall. In addition, the length, relationship to renal and iliac arteries can be readily assessed.

CT SIGNS OF IMPENDING RUPTURE

Patients with abdominal aortic aneurysm may present with chronic pain from impending rupture of enlarging abdominal aortic aneurysm. Aneurysm size is the most accurate positive predictive factor in determining the risk for rupture.

It has been shown that in patients with aneurysm larger than 5 cm in diameter, the aneurysm will rupture within 5 years of detection. Also an increase of 1 cm or more in the diameter of abdominal aortic aneurysm over the past 6 months is sign for impending rupture.[4]

The signs of impending rupture on CT are:[5]

1. The high attenuation crescent sign → This is the result of hemorrhage within the mural thrombus or wall of the aneurysm and may represent the first sign of rupture (Figure 9.1).
2. The draped aorta sign → This occurs when an area in the posterior wall of the aortic aneurysm is not identified and is closely apposed to the spine.
3. Focal discontinuity of the intimal calcification.

CT SIGNS OF RUPTURED ABDOMINAL AORTIC ANEURYSM

The helical CT signs of ruptured abdominal aortic aneurysm include retroperitoneal hematoma (Figure 9.2A) and extravasation of intravenous contrast. Hemorrhage is most often seen into the retroperitoneum involving the perirenal spaces. CT scan not only helps in detecting signs of rupture, it can also depict active bleeding, help localize the exact site of bleeding (Figure 9.2B), extension of the aneurysm into the common, external and internal iliac arteries. It can show the presence and extent of mural thrombus and the relationship of the renal arteries to the aneurysm. This added information is important for the choice of treatment/surgical planning.

TYPE B AORTIC DISSECTION

Acute type B aortic dissection is a potentially life-threatening condition and must be diagnosed and treated

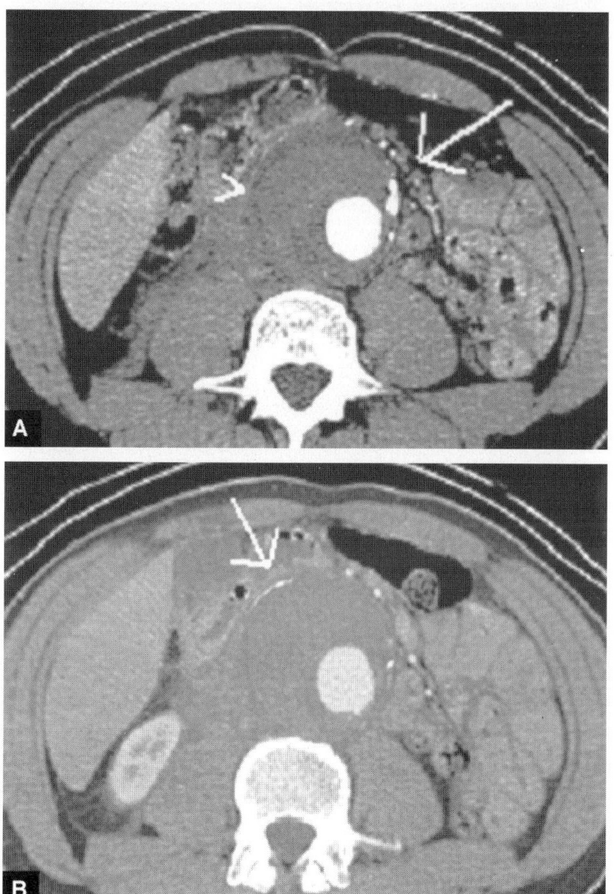

FIGURES 9.1A and B: Patient with history of abdominal aortic aneurysm, presenting with acute abdominal pain. (A,B) Axial scan with intravenous contrast showing a moderate sized abdominal aortic aneurysm(Large arrow) and the presence of curvilinear hyperdensity within its lumen (small arrow) , "the high attenuation crescent sign." The 'crescent sign' represents hemorrhage within the mural thrombus or wall of the aneurysm and may represent the first sign of rupture.

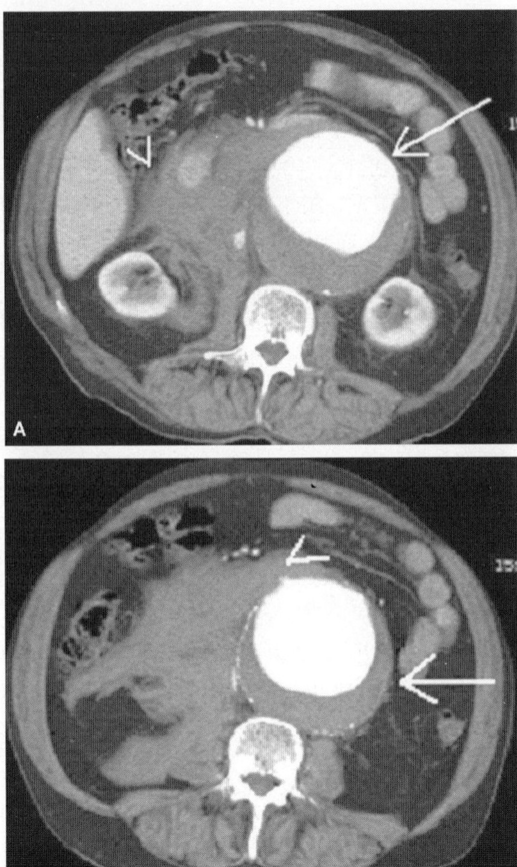

FIGURES 9.2A and B: Patient with history of abdominal aortic aneurysm, presenting with severe abdominal pain and suspected rupture. (A) axial scans with intravenous contrast showing a large abdominal aortic aneurysm.(large arrow) with extensive periaortic hematoma extending to the right pararenal space. (B) Again seen is a large abdominal aortic aneurysm.(large arrow) with extensive periaortic hematoma. Note the indistinct anterior wall with a niche of contrast (small arrow), likely representing the site of active bleed

early. Type B dissection originates distal to the origin of the left subclavian artery and extends caudally to the bifurcation/iliac arteries. Distal extension into the abdominal aorta and beyond is associated with branch vessel occlusion and associated ischemia or infarction in the involved vascular distribution. Patients may present with acute abdominal pain ranging from visceral ischemia, infarction or mesenteric ischemia.

Helical CT is now considered the screening modality of choice for aortic dissection.[6] The accuracy of helical CT is high with a sensitivity and specificity of nearly 100%.[6] Helical CT technique requires rapid (> 3 ml / sec) injection of intravenous contrast for optimal vascular opacification, thin 3 mm collimation and reformats.

The presence of a contrast filled double lumen with an intervening intimal flap is diagnostic of dissection (Figure 9.3).

Type B Aortic dissection is frequently complicated by abdominal branch vessel occlusion and may result in visceral or mesenteric ischemia (Figure 9.4).

Two types of branch vessel occlusion had been described by Sebastian et al:[6]

1. Static—wherein the intimal flap extends into the wall of the branch vessel.
2. Dynamic occlusion—wherein the flap prolapses across the branch vessel origin and covers the lumen like a curtain.

The frequency of branch vessel occlusion caused by dissection of abdominal aortic branches has been estimated as 27%.[7]

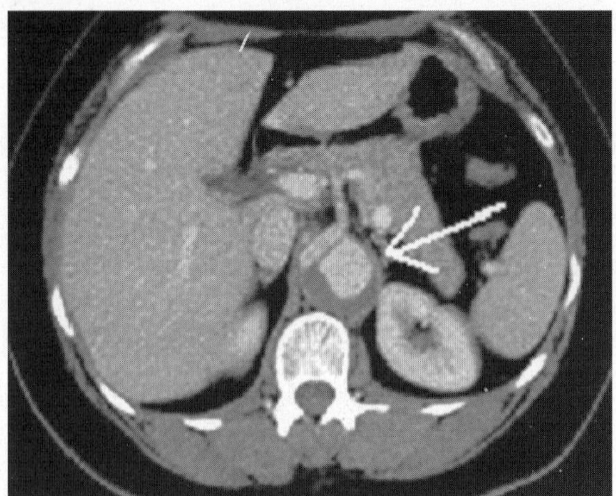

FIGURE 9.3: A case of type B aortic dissection. Axial scan at the level of the suprarenal aorta showing a type B dissection with the false lumen (arrow) filled with thrombus and larger in size .Note the SMA is arising anteriorly from the smaller true lumen

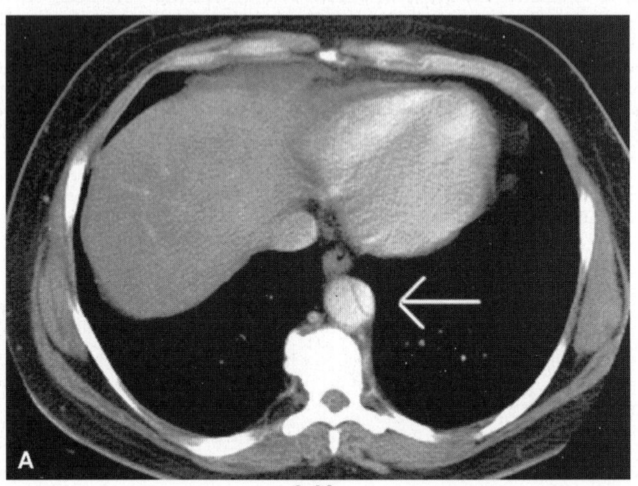

9.4A

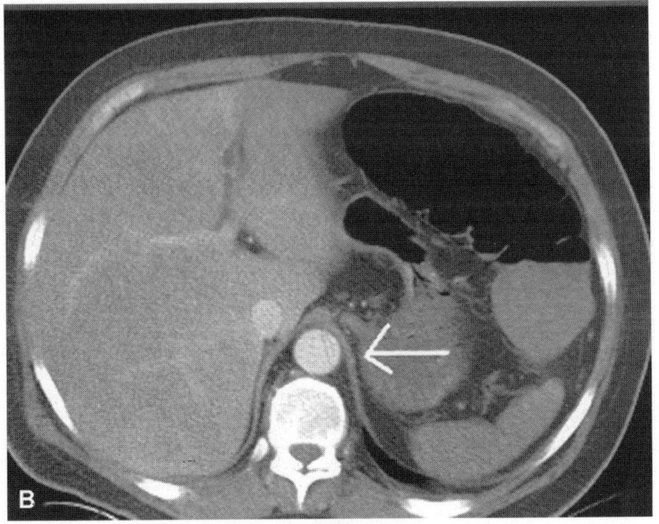

9.4B

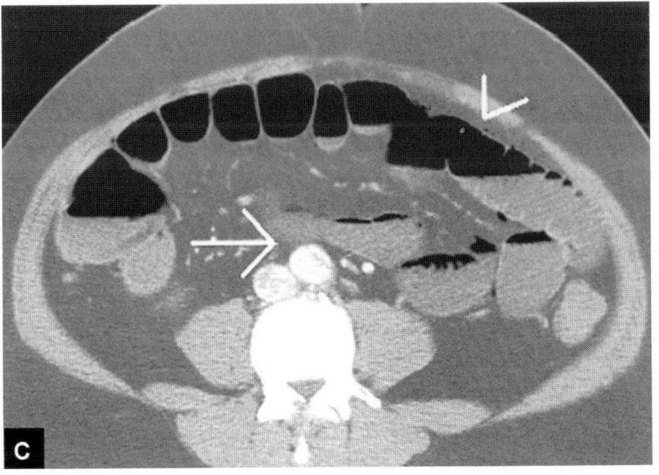

9.4C

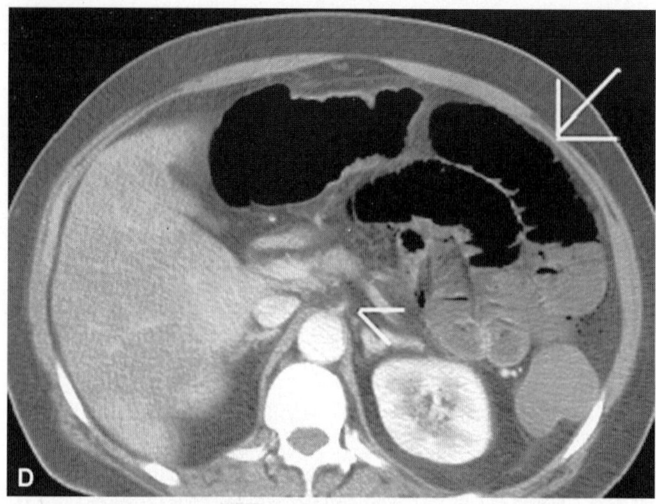

9.4D

FIGURES 9.4A to D: Patient with history of type B dissection presented with acute abdominal pain and suspected visceral ischemia. (A,B) Axial scans with iv contrast demonstrate type b dissection (arrows). (C) Caudal scans showing multiple dilated small bowel loops (small arrow) and dissection of the abdominal aorta (large arrow). (D) Scan at the level of the SMA showing poor enhancement of the proximal SMA (small arrow) and ischemic small bowel loops (large arrow)

In the presence of ischemia, the identification of the true and false lumen is important for treatment planning.

The following CT findings may favor a false lumen.

1. Beak sign:[7] Described by Page et al, The Beak sign is the cross-sectional imaging manifestation of the thin wedge of hematoma that forms at the interface between the propagating false lumen and the true lumen (Figure 9.5).

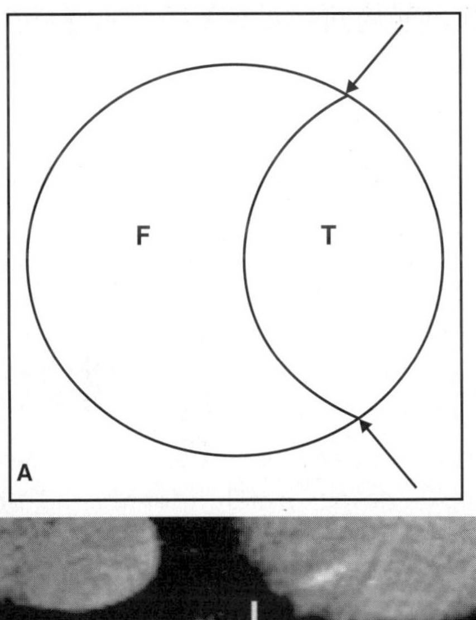

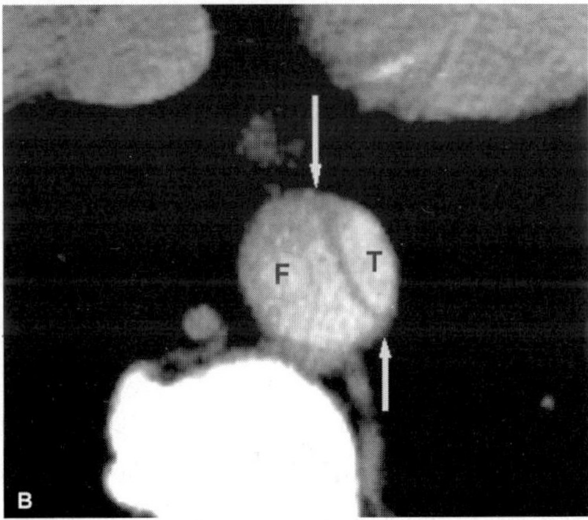

FIGURES 9.5A and B: The Beak sign in acute aortic dissection. (A) The illustrated line diagram demonstrates the true and false lumen with the appearance of a beak at the margin of true and false lumen (arrows). (B) Axial CT scan showing the presence of the larger false and smaller true lumen with beak sign (arrows). The Beak sign is the cross-sectional imaging manifestation of the thin wedge of hematoma that forms the interface between the propagating false lumen and the true lumen

2. Larger cross sectional area on contrast enhanced CT images
3. Less common identifiers are presence of intraluminal thrombus, presence of cobweb sign (i.e. thin linear intraluminal filling defects that represent ribbons of media that are incompletely sheared off by the dissection).

Features indicating a true lumen are:

1. A smaller cross sectional area on contrast enhanced CT images
2. Presence of outer wall and eccentric flap calcification

Thus CT can accurately identify the presence of dissection, the differentiation of true and false lumen and the presence of branch vessel occlusion and its sequale.

INTRA-ABDOMINAL HEMORRHAGE

Acute abdominal hemorrhage may occur in the bowel, mesentery, retroperitoneum, or abdominal muscles and patients may present with symptoms of an acute abdomen. Patients with significant bleeding may have declining hematocrit and hypotension. Early detection and treatment is essential to prevent mortality. CT scan is an ideal modality to detect intra-abdominal hemorrhage and also to detect any active site of hemorrhage.

Initially, unenhanced scans are obtained to detect a hyperdense hematoma. Later intravenous contrast material may be used to identify an active site of

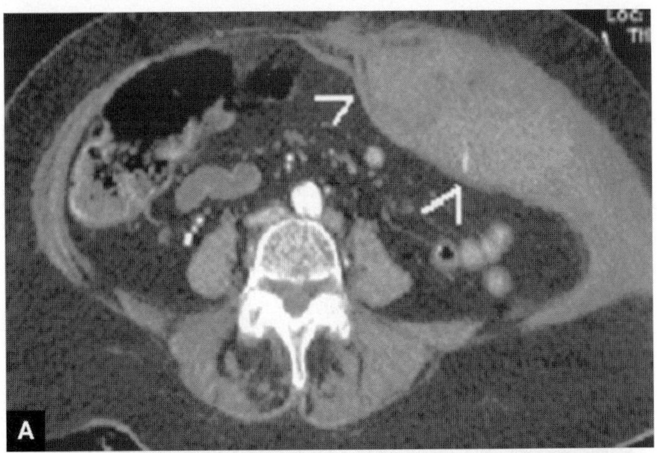

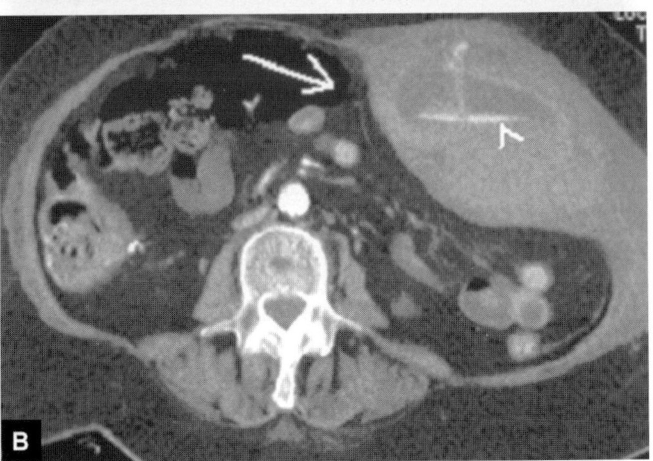

FIGURES 9.6A and B: Patient with history of anticoagulant therapy and severe abdominal pain. (A) Axial scans with intravenous contrast showing a large left rectus sheath hematoma (small arrows). (B) Another section showing the large left rectus sheath hematoma with active bleeding and hematocrit level (small arrow) very commonly seen with patients on anticoagulants

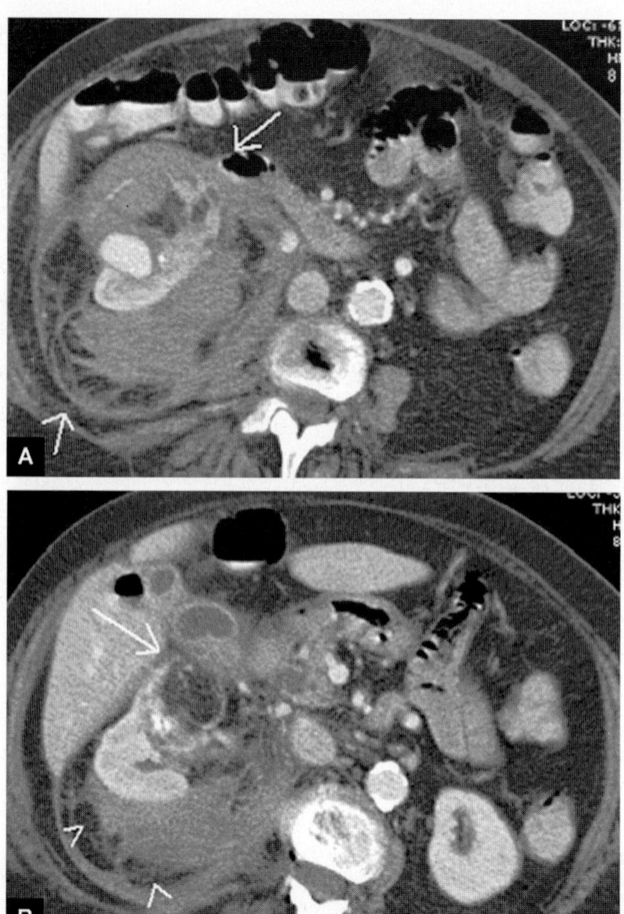

FIGURES 9.7A and B: Patient presenting with severe right-sided abdominal pain. (A) There is extensive right perinephric hematoma (arrows). (B) Axial scan showing extensive perinephric hematoma (small arrows), note a fat density lesion in the upper pole of right Kidney (large arrow) representing an angiomyolipoma, which caused spontaneous hemorrhage

hemorrhage and provide a useful guide for subsequent angiographic embolization.[8]

Spontaneous hemorrhage is common in patients who have received anticoagulant drug therapy.[9] It may occur spontaneously or result from minor trauma and affect any organ system Bleeding may occur into the rectus sheath (Figure 9.6), psoas muscle, the gut or from the kidneys. Occasionally, spontaneous renal hemorrhage may occur in the perinephric space or subcapsular region, most commonly in cases of renal cell carcinoma, angiomyolipomas (Figure 9.7) or post-lithotripsy.

POINTS TO REMEMBER

1. Vascular emergencies are life-threatening events and early diagnosis is essential to prevent mortality.
2. Look for early signs of impending rupture of abdominal aortic aneurysm like high attenuation crescent, discontinuous intimal calcification.
3. Branch vessel occlusion is a complication of type B dissection. Identification of true and false lumen is important for treatment planning.

REFERENCES

1. Bengtsson HK, Bergquist D. Ruptured abdominal aortic aneurysm: a population based study. J Vasc Surgery 1993; 18: 74-80.
2. Lederle FA, Johnson GR, Wilson SE, et al. Rupture rate of large abdominal aortic aneurysm in patients refusing or unfit for elective repair. JAMA 2002; 287: 2968-72.

3. Costello P. Gaa J. Spiral CT angiography of abdominal aortic aneurysm. Radiographics 1995; 15: 397-406.
4. Siegel CL, Cohan RH. CT of abdominal aortic aneurysm. AJR AM J Roentgenal 1994; 163: 17-29.
5. Mehard WB, Heiken JP, Sicard GA. High attenuating crescent in abdominal aortic aneurysm wall at CT: a sign of acute or impending rupture. Radiology 1994; 192: 359-62.
6. Sebastia C. Pallisa E, Quiroga S, Alvarez-Castells A. Dominquez R. Evangelista A. Aortic dissection: diagnosis and follow up with helical CT. Radiographics 1999; 19: 45-60.
7. Le Page MA, Quint LE, Sonnad SS, Deeb GM, Williams DM. Aortic dissection: CT features that distinguish true lumen from fasle lumen. AJR AMJ Roentgenal 2001; 177: 207-11.
8. Lane MJ, Katz DS, Shah RA, Rubin GD, Jeffrey RB Jr. Active arterial contrast extravasation on helical CT of the abdomen, pelvis, and chest. AJR 1998; 171: 679-85.
9. Pretorius ES, Fishman EK, Zinreich SJ. CT of hemorrhagic complications of anti-coagulant therapy. J Comput Assist Tomography 1997; 21: 44-51.

Chapter 10

Miscellaneous

MISCELLANEOUS ACUTE INTRA-ABDOMINAL PATHOLOGIES

There are a variety of miscellaneous acute intra-abdominal conditions that have a self limiting course and can be managed conservatively. However the clinical presentations are non-specific and can mimic appendicitis, cholecystitis or diverticulitis and surgery may in fact be advocated if accurate diagnosis is not made. Non-invasive diagnosis plays an important role in the diagnosis and prevents unnecessary surgeries.

In this chapter, we will discuss the CT appearances and diagnosis of the rare but clinically important causes of acute abdominal conditions.

EPIPLOIC APPENDAGITIS

Appendices epiploicae are pedunculated adipose structures protruding from the external surface of the colon. They extend from the cecum to the rectosigmoid junction. They are normally not visible on CT scans because they blend with the surrounding fat. Each of them is supplied by one to two small end arteries from the vasa recta of the colon and is drained by a vein. Because of their tortuous vascular supply, pedunculated shape and excessive mobility, they are prone to torsion and resultant ischemia or hemorrhagic infarction.[1]

Epiploic appendagitis is a rare inflammatory and ischemic condition that results from torsion or spontaneous venous thrombosis of one of the appendices epiploicae. Patients may present with sudden, severe focal abdominal pain in one of the lower quadrant and can mimic appendicitis or diverticulitis.

Non-invasive diagnosis is important as epiploic appendagitis is self-limiting and management is conservative.[2] However diagnosis is difficult clinically and surgery may be indicated.

CT Findings are Usually Diagnostic[3,4]

The CT findings include (Figures 10.1 and 10.2):

1. An oval paracolonic fatty mass surrounded by mesenteric stranding.
2. Well circumscribed hyper-attenuating rim surrounding the mass, represent the inflamed visceral peritoneum.
3. Sometimes a central high-attenuation "dot" representing an engorged or thrombosed vein can be identified within the inflamed appendage.

The other findings include mild-local reactive thickening of the adjacent colonic wall. However, the paracolonic inflammatory changes are disproportionately more severe than the bowel wall thickening.

OMENTAL INFARCTION

The omentum is a double layer of peritoneum that extends from the greater curvature of the stomach and drapes over the transverse colon (Figure 10.3).[5] The blood supply of the greater omentum is by the right and left gastroepiploic arteries.

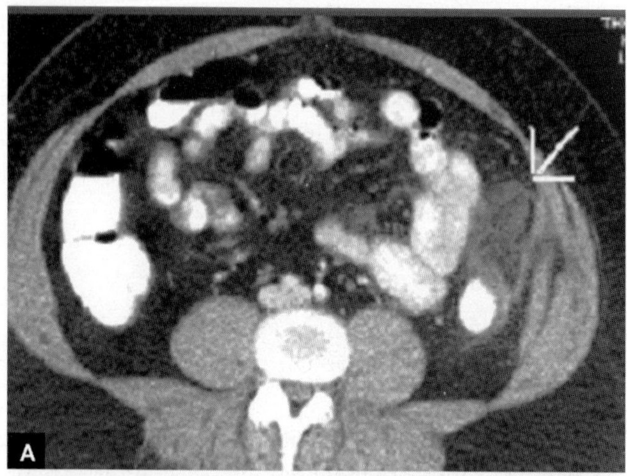

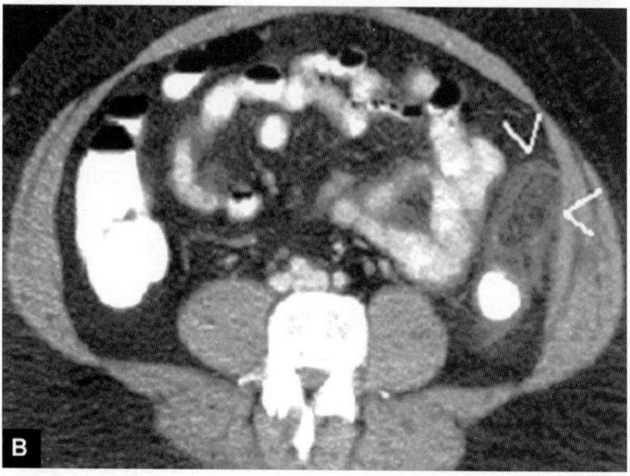

FIGURES 10.1A and B: Patient presenting with acute left lower quadrant pain and suspected diverticulitis. (A,B) Axial scans demonstrating an ovoid pericolonic fat density lesion in the left flank (arrows) with surrounding fat stranding. Note there is no significant bowel wall thickening

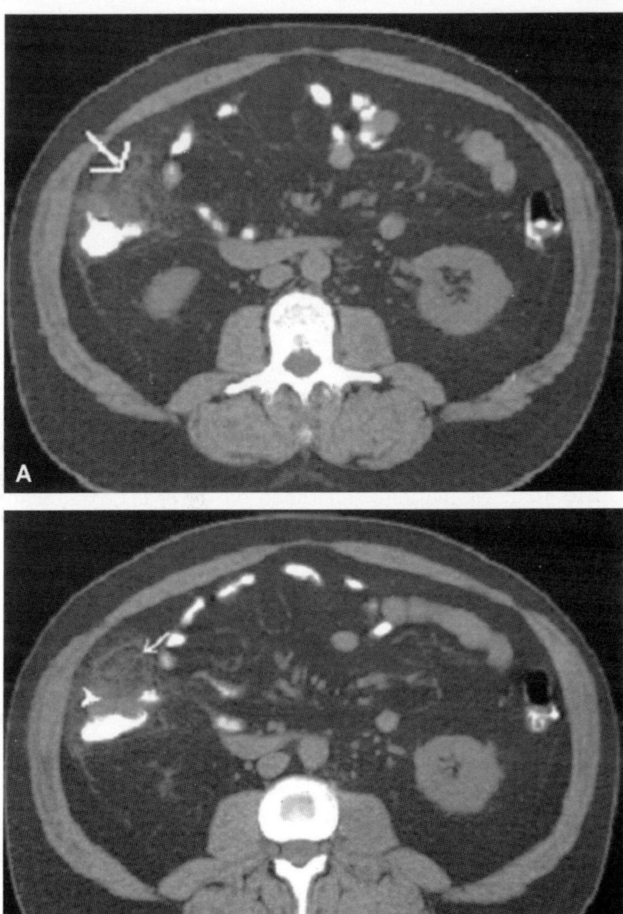

FIGURES 10.2A and B: Another example of appendigitis epiploica in a patient with right lower quadrant pain and suspected appendicitis. (A) Axial scan showing an ovoid pericolonic fat density lesion in the right lower quadrant (arrow). (B) Note there is minimal adjacent colonic wall thickening (arrow head), consistent with *Epiploic Appendagitis*

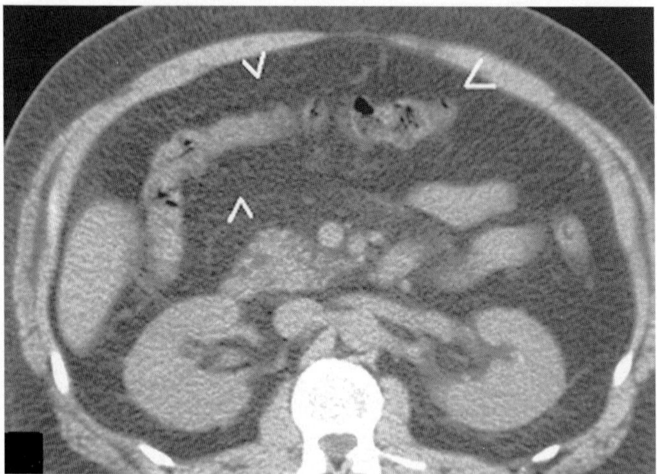

FIGURE 10.3: Normal omentum seen on CT scan. Axial scans demonstrating the normal omentum on CT scan (small arrows). The omentum is a double layer of peritoneum that extends from the greater curvature of the stomach and drape over the transverse colon

SEGMENTAL OMENTAL INFARCTION

On CT the greater omentum appears as a band of fatty tissue containing small vessels and is located anterior to the transverse colon.

Segmental omental infarction can occur, and is usually on the right side.[6] Risk factors include obesity and recent surgery. It can mimic appendicitis or cholecystitis clinically. It is usually self limiting and can be managed conservatively.

On CT the infarcted omentum appears as a large, high-attenuation fatty mass centered in the omentum (Figures 10.4 and 10.5). It may be close to the adjacent colon. Reactive bowel wall thickening may occur, but the

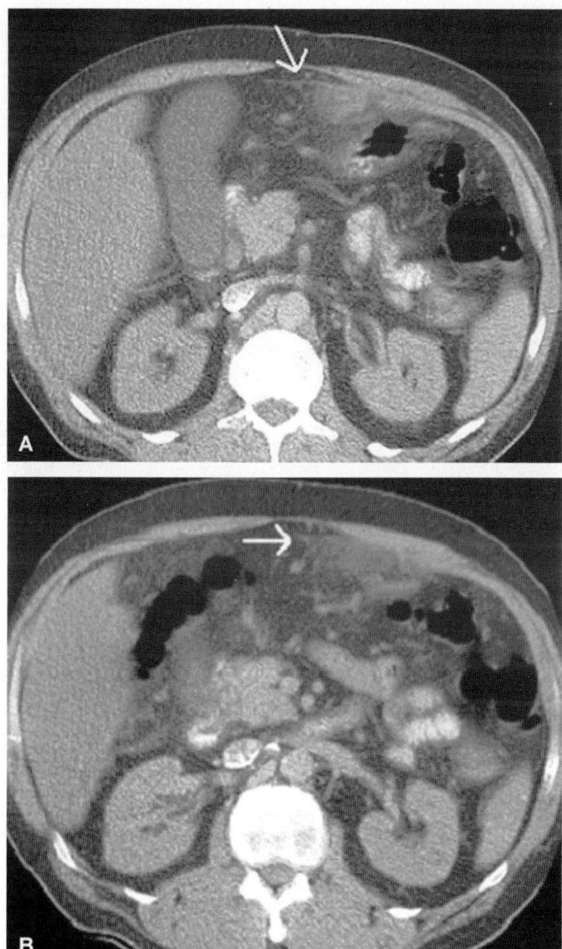

FIGURES 10.4A and B: Patient with history of upper mid-abdominal pain and suspected cholecystitis. (A,B) Axial scan of the upper abdomen showing an area of soft tissue density and surrounding fat stranding in the omentum (arrows) suggestive of omental infarction

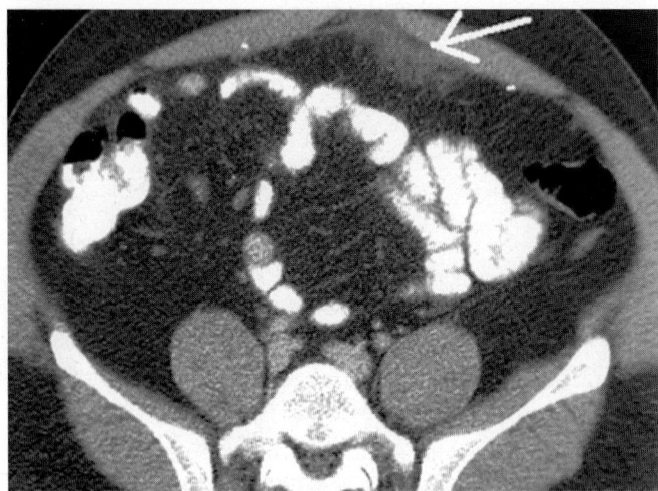

FIGURE 10.5: Another example of omental infarct. Axial scan demonstrating an area of increased density in the omentum (arrow) with fat stranding suggestive of omental infarct

inflammatory process is disproportionately more severe in the omentum. The CT appearance may be similar to epiploic appendagitis. The distinguishing features include-

Table 10.1[7]

Feature	Epiploic Appendagitis	Omental infarct
Location to colon	Always immediate adjacent to colon	Centered in omentum
Location of pain	RLQ, left lower quadrant	RLQ, RUQ
Central dot sign	Present	Absent
Hyperattenuated rim	Present	Absent

MESENTERIC PANNICULITIS

Mesenteric panniculitis is a rare idiopathic disorder characterized by nonspecific inflammation involving the fat of the small bowel mesentery.[8]

The clinical presentation is nonspecific and patients present with vague abdominal pain.

On CT scans, panniculitis characteristically manifests as a solitary well defined mass of inhomogeneous fatty tissue at the root of the jejunal mesentery (Figure 10.6A).

The fatty mass may engulf the superior mesenteric vessels without vascular narrowing. Well-defined soft tissue nodules usually less than 5 mm are seen scattered throughout the mass (Figure 10.6B). A distinctive hypo-attenuated fatty halo surrounds the nodules and vessels. This appearance helps in distinguishing mesenteric panniculitis from lymphoproliferative disorder and other causes of mesenteric adenopathy. Also a hyper-attenuating stripe surrounding the fatty mass may be suggestive of panniculitis. Thus, the characteristic CT appearance, location and the vague clinical presentation help in the diagnosis of this condition.

MESENTERIC ADENITIS

Detection of mesenteric lymphadenopathy on CT leads to an extensive and challenging differential diagnosis. The evaluation is based on size, number, location, and the appearance of the nodes. Inflammatory nodes in mesenteric adenitis are usually <10 mm in size,

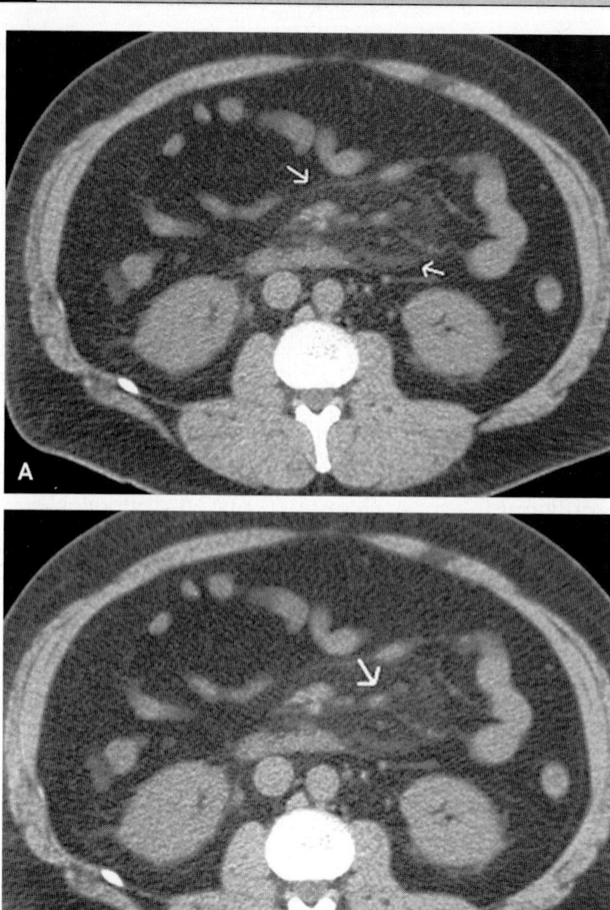

FIGURES 10.6A and B: Patient presented with mid abdominal pain and suspected pancreatitis. (A) Axial scan showing an area of increased fat density in the mid abdomen with well defined margins (arrows). (B) Note well-defined soft tissue nodules seen within the mass (arrow)

homogenously attenuating, clustered in the right lower quadrant, small bowel mesentery, or ventral to the psoas muscle.[9]

Mesenteric adenitis is a benign inflammation of the ileocolic lymph nodes. Mesenteric adenitis can be divided into primary and secondary types. Primary mesenteric adenitis has been defined as right-sided mesenteric lymphadenopathy without an identifiable acute inflammatory process or with only mild (< 5 mm) wall thickening of the terminal ileum. In most cases of primary mesenteric adenitis, an underlying infectious terminal ileitis is thought to be the cause.[10]

Secondary mesenteric adenitis is defined as lymphadenopathy associated with a detectable intra-abdominal inflammatory process.[11]

Primary mesenteric adenitis is more common in children than adults.

In patients with primary mesenteric adenitis, the clinical presentation is nonspecific (abdominal pain, fever and leukocytosis) and clinically may mimic appendicitis, infectious enterocolitis, diverticulitis, perforated cecal carcinoma, PID, renal stones and pyelonephritis.

On CT scan, the mesenteric lymph nodes are enlarged (> 5 mm) though usually less than 10 mm, clustered in the right lower quadrant (Figure 10.7A) and are of homogenous attenuation (criteria—at least 3 lymph nodes of >5 mm each). The appendix is normal and there may be mild thickening of terminal ileum usually < 5 mm (Figure 10.7B), also there may be inflammation in the surrounding mesentery (Figure 10.8).

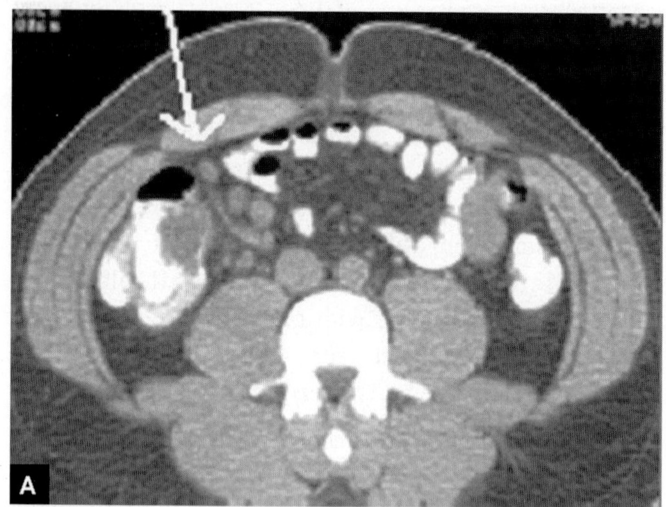

10.7A

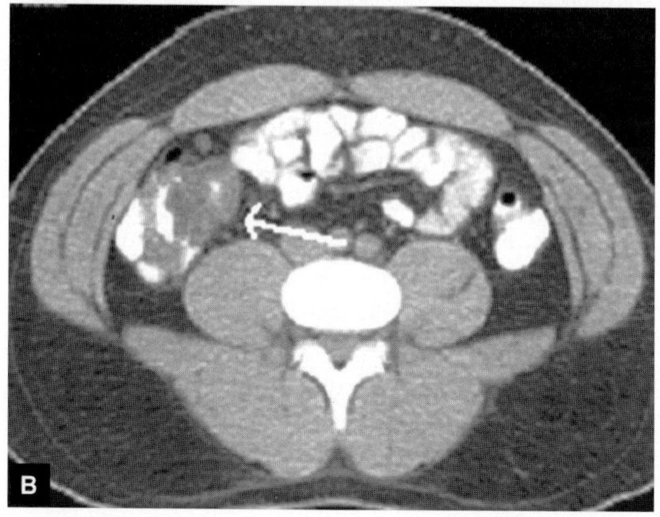

10.7B

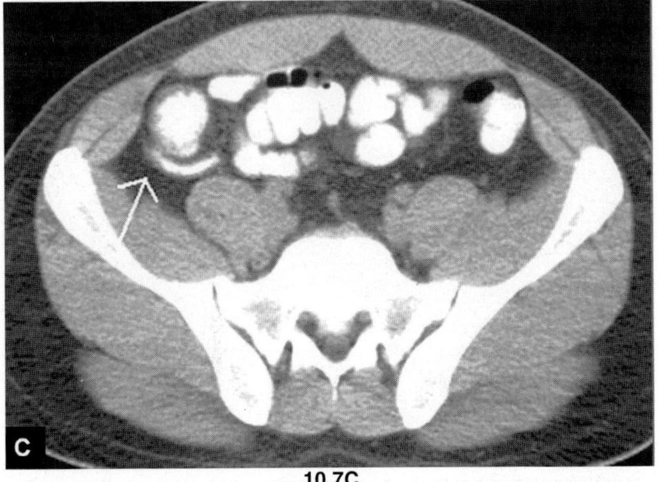

10.7C

FIGURES 10.7A to C: Patient with right lower quadrant pain and clinically suspected appendicitis. (A) Axial scan showing multiple enlarged mesenteric lymph nodes (arrow) in the right lower quadrant. (B) There is mild thickening of the terminal ileum (arrow). (C) Note the appendix is filled with oral contrast and within normal limits (arrow)

Rao et al[9] found primary mesenteric adenitis to be the second most common cause of right lower quadrant after appendicitis, accounting for 7% of the discharge diagnoses in adult and pediatric patients with clinical suspicion for appendicitis.

Thus, CT can therefore help differentiate primary mesenteric adenitis from the above-mentioned entities, allowing for a more accurate diagnosis and help patients avoid undergoing surgery.

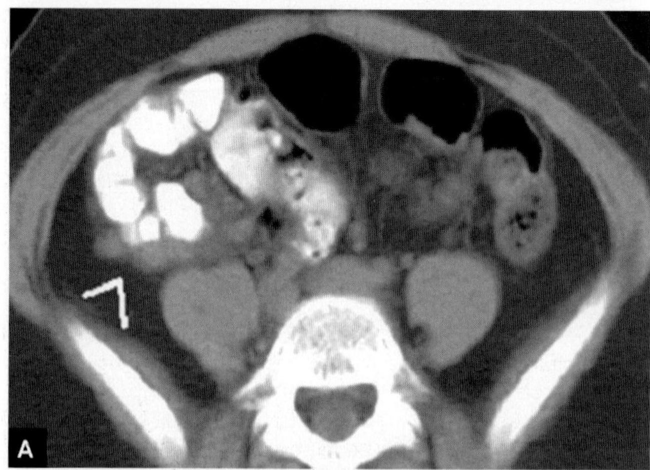

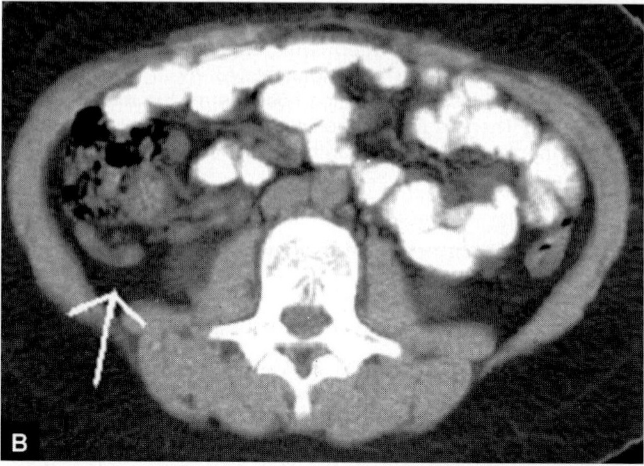

FIGURES 10.8A and B: Another example of mesenteric adenitis in a patient with right lower quadrant pain and clinically suspected appendicitis. (A) Axial scan showing multiple enlarged mesenteric lymph nodes (small arrow) in the right lower quadrant. (B) The appendix is of normal caliber (large arrow)

REFERENCES

1. Ghahremani GG, white EM ,Hoff FL, Gore RM Miller JW, Christ ML. Appendices epiploicae of colon: Radiologic and pathologic features. Radiographics 1992; 12; 59-77.
2. Legome EL, Belton AL, Murray RE, Rao. PM, Novelline RA, Epiploic appendagitis: the emergency department presentation. J Emerg med 2002; 22;9-13.
3. Rao PM, Wittenberg J, Lowrason JN. Primary epiploic appendagitis: evolutionary changes in CT appearance. Radiology 1997;204:713-717.
4. Torres GM, Abbitt PL, Weeks M. CT Manifestation of infarcted epiploic appendages of the colon. Abdom Imaging 1994; 19: 449-50.
5. Somepayeac SW, Mindelzun RE, Silverman PM Sze R. The greater omentum. AJR roentgenol 1997;168:683-7.
6. Epstein LI, lempke RE. Primary idiopathic segmental infarction of the greater omentum: Case report and collective review of the literature. Ann Surg 1968; 167;437-43.
7. Van Breda Vriesman AC, Lohle, PN, Corekamp EG, Puylaert JB. Infarction of omentum and epiploic appendage: diagnosis epidemiology and natural history. Eur Radiol 1999; 9: 1886-92.
8. Daskalogiannaki N. Voloudaki A, Prassopoulos P, et al. CT evaluation of mesenteric panniculitis: Prevalence and associated disease. AJR Am J Roentgenol 2000; 147:427-31.
9. Rao PM, Rhea JT, Novelline RA, CT diagnosis of mesenteric adenitis. Radiology 1997;202:145-9.
10. Puylert JB. Mesenteric adenitis and acute terminal ileitis: US evaluation using graded compression. Radiology 1986;161: 691-5.
11. Al-Kawas FH, Murgo A. Foshag L, Shiels W. Lymphadenopathy in iliac disease: not always a sign of lymphoma. AmJ Gastroenterol 1988; 83: 303.

INDEX